PRAISE FOR
ASHKENAZI HERBALISM

"A significant contribution to Jewish studies—Cohe　　　　　　　. successfully resolved the mystery of Ashkenazi herbal traditions."

—MAREK TUSZEWICKI,
deputy director of the Institute of Jewish Studies,
Jagiellonian University in Kraków and author of
A Frog Under the Tongue

"Cohen and Siegel have offered us a priceless jewel: a historical document of Jewish herbal heritage that blazes with life, revealing vital roots long buried in obscurity. . . . Ashkenazi Herbalism is an important addition to the canon of herbal literature, bequeathing to us a tradition of herbal practice that, but for their efforts, would have remained lost to the world."

—JUDITH BERGER,
writer, herbalist, and author of *Herbal Rituals*

"A delightfully written and highly original work that sheds new light on a woefully understudied aspect of Eastern European Jewish folk culture. The common stereotype of shtetl life is that Jews were cut off from the natural environment that surrounded them. Cohen's and Siegel's pioneering book reveals, by contrast, some of the ways in which Ashkenazi Jews in the Pale of Settlement and neighboring regions were deeply embedded in their local ecologies and possessed a rich heritage of herbal practices and knowledge."

—NATHANIEL DEUTSCH,
professor of history at the University of California,
Santa Cruz and author of *The Jewish Dark Continent*

"Meticulously researched and well written, Ashkenazi Herbalism is the fascinating account of the healing traditions and herbal medicine practiced by Eastern European Jews. . . . A brilliant work that captures an important but long-ignored facet of traditional herbal healing practices."

—ROSEMARY GLADSTAR,
herbalist and author of *Rosemary Gladstar's Medicinal Herbs*
and *Rosemary Gladstar's Herbal Recipes for Vibrant Health*

"Reading Ashkenazi Herbalism *is like finding a family heirloom you thought had been lost forever. . . . This book, full of rigorously researched ethnobotany and shtetl magic, is an answered prayer for those of us who have longed to reconnect with Ashkenazi folk healing traditions.*"

—DORI MIDNIGHT,
community healer, herbalist, and educator who incorporates
traditional healing practices and social justice in her work

"Ashkenazi Herbalism *explores the local and exotic plants Eastern European Jews used as medicine. After a thorough discussion of Jewish medical practitioners, especially female folk healers, it draws on a wide range of sources to look at how plants—alphabetically from aloe to nutmeg to violets—were used in the Russian Jewish Pale of Settlement compared to other times and places.*"

—GABRIELLA SAFRAN,
Eva Chernov Lokey Professor in Jewish Studies at
Stanford University and author of *Wandering Soul*

"Ashkenazi Herbalism *fascinates the reader with its deep detective work and thorough research of a healing tradition that was mostly lost by the horror and genocide of the Second World War, which destroyed Jewish communities and culture throughout Europe. . . . Thankfully, the authors have captured the Ashkenazi healing traditions that were practiced by itinerant Kabbalists, feldshers, and midwives so that these precious remnants of knowledge are not forgotten. Whether you are an avid herbalist, history buff, or plant lover, you'll find something in this book to satisfy your soul. What a gift to us all.*"

—PHYLLIS D. LIGHT, MA,
herbalist and author of *Southern Folk Medicine*

"[Cohen's] *deep dive into the past to bring forth the plant knowledge once practiced by the Ashkanazi people is a great contribution to future generations.*"

—PAM FISCHER,
executive director of the Berkeley Herbal Center

ASHKENAZI
HERBALISM

ASHKENAZI
HERBALISM

REDISCOVERING THE
HERBAL TRADITIONS OF
EASTERN EUROPEAN JEWS

DEATRA COHEN

AND

ADAM SIEGEL

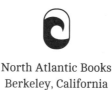

North Atlantic Books
Berkeley, California

Published by
North Atlantic Books
Huichin, unceded Ohlone land
aka Berkeley, California

Cover design by Rob Johnson
Book design by Happenstance Type-O-Rama

Printed in the United States of America

Ashkenazi Herbalism: Rediscovering the Herbal Traditions of Eastern European Jews is sponsored and published by North Atlantic Books, an educational nonprofit based in the unceded Ohlone land Huichin (*aka* Berkeley, CA) that collaborates with partners to develop cross-cultural perspectives; nurture holistic views of art, science, the humanities, and healing; and seed personal and global transformation by publishing work on the relationship of body, spirit, and nature.

North Atlantic Books' publications are distributed to the US trade and internationally by Penguin Random House Publisher Services. For further information, visit our website at www.northatlanticbooks.com.

MEDICAL DISCLAIMER: The following information is intended for general information purposes only. Individuals should always see their health care provider before administering any suggestions made in this book. Any application of the material set forth in the following pages is at the reader's discretion and is their sole responsibility.

Library of Congress Cataloging-in-Publication Data
Names: Cohen, Deatra, 1964– author. | Siegel, Adam, 1966– author.
Title: Ashkenazi herbalism : rediscovering the herbal traditions of eastern
  European Jews / Deatra Cohen and Adam Siegel.
Description: Berkeley, California : North Atlantic Books, [2021] |
  Includes bibliographical references and index. | Summary: "A rediscovery
  of the forgotten legacy of the Jewish medicinal plant healers who
  thrived in eastern Europe's Pale of Settlement, from the Middle Ages
  through the modern era"—Provided by publisher.
Identifiers: LCCN 2020042445 (print) | LCCN 2020042446 (ebook) | ISBN
  9781623175443 (trade paperback) | ISBN 9781623175450 (ebook)
Subjects: LCSH: Medicinal plants. | Materia medica, Vegetable. |
  Herbs—Therapeutic use. | Jews—Medicine.
Classification: LCC QK99.A1 C64 2021 (print) | LCC QK99.A1 (ebook) | DDC
  581.6/34—dc23
LC record available at https://lccn.loc.gov/2020042445
LC ebook record available at https://lccn.loc.gov/2020042446

4 5 6 7 8 9 KPC 25 24 23 22

THIS BOOK IS DEDICATED TO
JEROME SIEGEL (1933–2020)

CONTENTS

PREFACE

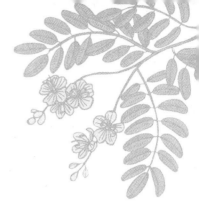

ON THE SURFACE, HERBALISM, OR HERBAL MEDICINE, seems a simple enough concept. It's the reliance upon plant medicine to heal a body from disease, with an eye toward returning that body to its natural state of balance. But herbalism is a much more complex practice than one might assume.

According to the American Herbalists Guild:

> *Herbal medicine is the art and science of using herbs for promoting health and preventing and treating illness. It has persisted as the world's primary form of medicine since the beginning of time, with a written history more than 5000 years old. While the use of herbs in America has been overshadowed by dependence on modern medications in the last 100 years, 75% of the world's population still rely primarily upon traditional healing practices, most of which is herbal medicine.[1]*

Human reliance on the medicinal properties of plants is ancient and worldwide, but as universal as our connection may be, our ways of working with the plants can vary. One reason for this is environmental: every part of Earth is distinct, with its own indigenous fauna and flora that are each dependent on their unique natural surroundings and each other. The plants and animals that settle and evolve in one region become accustomed to that region's local weather conditions, soil composition, and all the other organisms and creatures with whom they share their habitat. In this way, for example, native peoples living near the equator are familiar with completely different circumstances than those who call the Arctic home. These two distinct ecosystems provide very different life experiences—and challenges—for the humans and other living organisms who settle there.

But humans are not the only ones who endure the conditions of our domains. Plants also need to maintain vitality within the dynamic conditions of their environment. To overcome the hardships they've encountered, plants have learned how best to persist in the face of environmental adversity. It's these verdant secrets of survival that have drawn humans and other organisms to the flora that flourish in our midsts. Through our contacts with the plant world, we've learned not only how to survive over countless generations but also how to thrive on this tumultuous planet we call home.

When I began studying herbalism, the program where I was enrolled encouraged students to get to know our own ancestral healing practices.* This idea isn't unique to any particular herbal school; most if not all herbalists are curious about their own ancestors' traditional practices and often look there for inspiration and guidance.

When you consider our ancestors' relationship with plants for healing and sustenance, over thousands of years, it makes sense that our bodies, on a physical level at the very least, would have traces of the essences that contributed so much to our well-being.

In fact, humans have relied on plants for almost all of our basic needs: food, drink, housing, utensils, tools, clothing, energy, companionship, warmth. Plants have even been the subject of some of our most memorable stories. Who doesn't remember the three magic beans that grew overnight into the stalk Jack climbed up into the clouds to find the giant? Or, in more contemporary literature, the endless sea of red poppies that lulled Dorothy and her friends into sleep on their way to see the Wizard? We've had a long and intimate relationship with the plant world, and whether our minds are conscious of it or not, our bodies seem to remember more than they let on. Examples of stored memories might come in the form of an allergic reaction to strawberries or peanuts, salivation in response to the taste of any bitter herb, or, in my case, a vaporous memory conjured in my forties when I experienced the scent of a linden tree in bloom for the first time. To my knowledge I'd never come across this kind of tree before, and yet as soon as I was aware of its fragrance, I felt like I'd come home. On a purely

---

* The first-person singular is used by Deatra throughout to describe her impressions and experiences in researching and writing this book.

visceral level, we're already familiar with many of the plants we encounter, and our individual interactions with them are based on long-forgotten connections waiting to be reawakened.

Having been a professional librarian for many years, I was looking forward to researching what I assumed would be a good-sized collection of resources devoted to the medicinal plant knowledge of the people I call my ancestors. Both sides of my family are Ashkenazi from the Pale of Settlement. My father's family emigrated to the United States and Canada in the early twentieth century from what today is Ukraine, specifically the cities of Kiev and Cherkassy. Both of my mother's parents were from the same region of Poland; one branch of that family can be traced back to their town's founding in the early eighteenth century, where they stayed put until the outbreak of the Second World War.

One might assume that Ashkenazim, who have a well-documented history in Eastern Europe's Pale of Settlement (the Pale) dating at least as far back as the Middle Ages, would have an exhaustive and distinguished canon dedicated to their healing practices, which would, no doubt, include the reliance upon plant medicine. But that assumption couldn't be further from the truth.

Once I started my research, I was at first surprised and then shocked at the complete absence of any information whatsoever on herbalism in any Ashkenazi communities of the Pale. And I wasn't alone in my discovery, or lack thereof. A few other students in my class who were of similar background also came up empty-handed. Out of frustration, one of us joked, "Well, at least we have chicken soup!" She was just as amazed as I that there was literally nothing else to be found, but she consoled herself with the belief that of course older generations had relied on plant medicine. And if they hadn't, it was probably because of religious restrictions.

I mulled all this over. Even though I hadn't been raised religiously and know next to nothing about Judaism, it seemed doubtful that any religion, no matter how strict, would keep the people from taking care of themselves. What little I did know was that the Jews had endured countless hardships and, despite these, had survived for thousands of years. There must have been a little bit of help from the natural world they lived in, and this would have included any medicinal plants in the vicinity.

Falling back on my librarian roots, I figured someone somewhere in the last century must have conducted an ethnobotanical study of the Ashkenazi people of the Pale. It seemed natural that an objective third party would have facilitated a basic survey of such a well-known population.[*]

But even a thorough search of the ethnobotanical literature proved fruitless. Information I assumed would be abundant was nonexistent. My husband, who speaks and reads multiple languages, many of them relevant for this research, foraged through multiple sources of every possible linguistic angle regarding the subject. It eventually became undeniably clear that not only was an ethnobotanical survey of Eastern Europe's Ashkenazim nonexistent, but there was next to nothing published describing the healers themselves who would have applied the medicinal plant knowledge.

I could not accept this turn of events. For better or worse, my past profession dogged me and I became more relentless in my mission to find evidence of Ashkenazi herbalism. Was this the ancestors urging me on? Who knows. But I do know that I didn't want to feel like an herbal interloper, forever having to refer to other peoples' traditions, never knowing what plant knowledge my own grandparents had relied on. I was certain that if I continued searching I would eventually stumble on some evidence I knew was out there.

My persistence led to more than a few dead ends, but every so often I came across tantalizing fragments of an Ashkenazi herbal past that were like a diaspora in their own right. I occasionally had the minor breakthrough, like the night I was half-heartedly searching for images of healers in a database dedicated to the Holocaust. Instead of portraits, I found a photograph of what looked like a vintage milk bottle. When I zoomed in to get a better view, its intact label hinted at a fascinating and completely unexpected story. This was a bottle of "bitters," a liqueur infused with medicinal herbs, such as gentian, for digestive health. Later I found that these aperitifs were common in Ashkenazi communities both in and outside the Pale.

---

[*] According to the *Merriam-Webster* dictionary, *ethnobotany*—which became an academic discipline in the 1890s—focuses its attention on the plant lore of Indigenous cultures and also the systematic study of such lore.

Another image search for the elusive folk healers of the Pale led me to sources I might not have found otherwise. One of these is a catalog to an exhibition. It features photographs taken in the early twentieth-century towns and villages of the Pale during the An-Sky expeditions. Who was An-Sky and why is his work important to discovering the herbal legacy of Eastern Europe's Ashkenazim of the early twentieth century? An-Sky's ethnographic work is one of many sources I wove together to bring the story of Ashkenazi herbalism into better focus in the pages ahead.

Another source was an ethnobotanical field study of sorts undertaken by the Soviet government between the world wars in an attempt to locate inexpensive medicines after domestic supplies had been depleted. The author of the study managed to bring the original research with her to the United States after the Second World War and, through government agencies that existed at the time, had an excerpt of that field work translated into English and published as part of a Cold War series on Eastern Europe. This document ostensibly covered the Eastern Europe of my ancestors; however, its vague language at first distracted me from understanding its true contents.

There was something undeniably mysterious about this book, but its presentation made it difficult to interpret. On the surface it looks like an outdated government document that easily could have been the victim of a vigorous weeding project at any public library. For some reason still unknown to me, I decided to more closely explore the data it so innocuously presented.

While the author never truly identifies the folk healers interviewed for the study, one of the book's appendices lists many of the towns that were targeted for the surveys. On a whim I started to investigate the towns identified, and almost immediately it became clear that most of these were located along the Dnieper River in what is present-day Ukraine. A large percentage of these were on the right bank. They were Ashkenazi towns and villages (Yiddish: *shtetlekh* and *derfer*) of the Pale of Settlement.

Once I started to untangle the information the book presented, a very unexpected trail of clues emerged. To make certain I was on the right path, I spent the next six months deciphering the book's anecdotal data. Eventually I had to tape together pieces of graph paper to make a huge table so I could accurately plot the information scattered throughout the document. From there I created a spreadsheet that I could more easily search and sort. I wanted both to get a better understanding of the hidden content I had inadvertently discovered and also to find any patterns that might emerge from it.

After I finished all of this, the puzzle pieces fell into place. Not only had I stumbled onto the herbs known by Eastern Europe's Ashkenazi healers at the turn of the twentieth century, but I had also found the healers themselves. This is their story.

PART I
A History of Ashkenazi Folk Healers

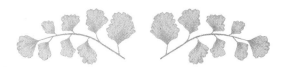

FROM TIME IMMEMORIAL, HUMANS HAVE LOOKED TO the natural world, which we always have been a part of, in order to heal ourselves. In this respect the Jews of Eastern Europe were no different from any other people. If anything, what set many Eastern European Jewish communities apart by the twentieth century was a reluctance to embrace the modern era and all the advantages promised by its technologies, including medicine. Had the Second World War not destroyed their communities, the natural healing traditions that had kept Eastern European Jews resilient for centuries would still be known today. Instead, this essential part of their history has been long obscured and, consequently, utterly forgotten by posterity. But who were the Eastern European Jews, and what evidence remains of their traditional healing practices?

To attempt to answer the latter question, we offer a brief sketch of folk medicine, Eastern European Jewry, the communities in which Eastern European (known for the most part as *Ashkenazi*) Jews lived, and what the written historical record reveals about their health practices and beliefs, in both "official" medicine (whether religious or secular) and folk medicine. We describe and discuss the different Jewish healers who treated Eastern European Jews (and their non-Jewish neighbors). And we contrast the worlds of men and women healers (again, whether religious or secular, and in official or folk medicine).

CHICKEN SOUP THEORY

Today the popular notion of healing among Ashkenazim is often reduced to "chicken soup," but Eastern European Jews have a highly complex medicinal tradition that dates back to the Hebrew Bible. The historical records of Jewish communities across many centuries and lands (the ancient Near East, the Islamic world, medieval Europe, etc.) reveal a rich variety of practices that include plant-based remedies. Oddly enough, if the researcher seeks out evidence of herbalism in modern Eastern European Jewish communities, the written record falls largely silent.

While many aspects of Ashkenazi life and culture have been thoroughly documented, researched, and examined, the majority of mainstream scholarship focusing on the history of Ashkenazi communities has almost entirely ignored the existence of traditional healers among the Ashkenazim; if discussed at all, folk healers have generally been portrayed as backward, ignorant, and foolish. Such dismissiveness is closely tied to the modern medical culture's interest in elevating its reputation among the general population by discounting premodern traditions and their practitioners and maligning healers lacking formal medical training as "superstitious," "quacks," and so forth.[2] Despite the longstanding and tireless efforts to "eradicate" their practices, however, Ashkenazi folk medicinal practitioners had an enduring presence in Eastern Europe for centuries, and they were an integral part of community well-being until deep into the twentieth century.[3]

One current authority, the *YIVO Encyclopedia of Jews in Eastern Europe*, tells readers that traditionally the Ashkenazi approach to health care made no distinction between what would now be considered "scientific" and "folk" medicines. While the entry reveals that Ashkenazim relied heavily on medicinal plants for their well-being right up until the destruction of European Jewry, it completely passes over which plants served as their familiar folk remedies.[4]

FOLK MEDICINE

The World Health Organization's website, in its section devoted to "Traditional, Complementary and Integrative Medicine," defines *folk medicine* as "the sum total of the knowledge, skills, and practices based on the theories, beliefs, and experiences indigenous to different cultures, whether explicable or not, used in the maintenance of health as well as in the prevention, diagnosis, improvement or treatment of physical and mental illness."[5]

Contemporary researchers expand this definition further, illuminating some areas where clinical Western medicine fears to tread: the folk healer is the catalyst whose medicine is to bring luck, calm evil spirits, or conjure love. Their expertise is often sought to restore order by pacifying evil spirits, removing states of dis-ease, and restoring harmony. Through the folk healer's work, a patient can be reintegrated into health and normality. In this way, the healer plays an elemental role in the social order of a culture, restoring the balance of collective community health.[6]

Because Eastern European Jews practiced folk medicine alongside Western medicine, if we want to better understand and appreciate the richness of their healing traditions, including their knowledge of medicinal plants, we'll have to look at both tradition and progress and embrace a more inclusive view.

PLANTS AND FOLK MEDICINE

Modern scientific literature discussing folk medicine relies on a binary that contrasts "herbal" and "magico-religious." *Herbal medicine* refers to healing through the application of plants, herbs, and other natural substances found locally.[7] It's self-evident that human beings all over the world have discovered, through direct experience and knowledge transmitted over thousands of years, the healing powers of the natural world around us.

By contrast *magico-religious medicine* means it relies on "nonmaterial" curative powers. The attribution of supernatural forces as causes of natural phenomena is a cultural universal that helps humans better understand their place in the cosmos. Supernatural forces provide an explanation for problems of all sorts, including sickness and environmental disasters. In order to restore natural balance or cure illness, humans have appealed to these forces by conjuring magic, reciting incantations, and performing rituals.

But herbal and magico-religious medicine have never been separate practices—they've always been intricately interwoven. In herbal medicine, a plant, or a specific part of a plant, might be understood to have healing powers. In magico-religious medicine, the same plant is known to have healing powers when it's applied to a wound if accompanied by the recitation of a prayer. Folk medicine practitioners have always understood the important connection between magic and herbal remedies. They believe that remedies work not only because of the plants and other substances they apply, but also through the power of an incantation and other scientifically inexplicable factors. In this way, the folk healer has been at once the restorer of balance and the symbol of the possibility of balance.[8]

In Eastern Europe, Ashkenazi Jews were one of many cultures whose folk medicine traditions embraced both herbal and magico-religious practices. All of the region's cultures contributed to a complex mélange of healing arts going back centuries, if not millennia. And, it might be surprising to learn, the folk healing practices of Ashkenazi Jews were so inextricably bound up with those of their neighbors that they often were virtually indistinguishable from one another.

BARRIERS TO DISCOVERING ASHKENAZI FOLK TRADITIONS

Yet even after we recognize these cultural, historical, and geographical inter-relations, the path to their medicinal plants still remains veiled in mystery. Why is this? For anyone interested in identifying both the healing methods and, more specifically, the herbs that were known to Eastern European Jews at the turn of the twentieth century, a number of barriers stand in the way of any significant discoveries. Information is piecemeal and often only available in one of a wide variety of languages, including Yiddish, Hebrew, Russian, Polish, Ukrainian, German, French, Hungarian, Latin, and Greek. Moreover, much of the mainstream scholarship on the history of Ashkenazi Jews has focused on narrow aspects of their communities, leaving considerable swaths of their legacy neglected and ignored. And finally, the deeply rooted culture of the Jews of Eastern Europe was utterly destroyed between 1939 and 1945. So in order to unearth the less-understood areas of their story, such as their herbal traditions, it's first necessary to re-examine some of what's currently believed about the cultures of health and sickness among the Ashkenazim.

THE ASHKENAZIM AND THE PALE OF SETTLEMENT

Toward the end of the first millennium, one wave of diaspora Jews whose origins lay in the Near East emerged in communities along the Rhine River in what is

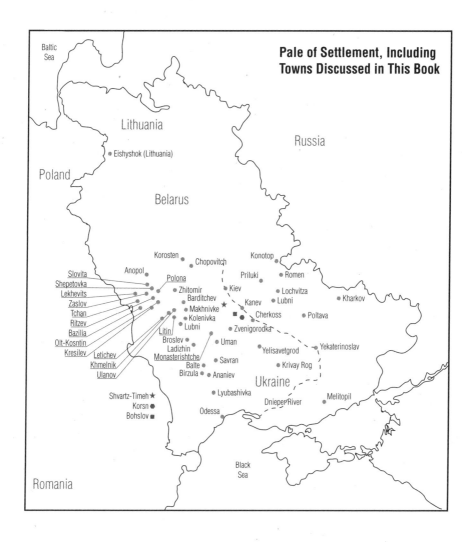

Pale of Settlement, Including
Towns Discussed in This Book

Baltic Sea

Lithuania

Russia

• Eishyshok (Lithuania)

Poland

Belarus

Korosten •   • Chopovitch   Konotop •
Slovita   Anopol •   Polona   Priluki •   • Romen
Shepetovka   • Zhitomir   • Kiev   • Lochvitza
Lekhevits   • Barditchev   Kanev • Lubni   • Kharkov
Zaslov   • Makhnivke   ★
Tchan   • Kolenivka   Cherkoss
Ritzev   • Lubni   • Poltava
Bazilia   Litin   • Zvenigorodka
Olt-Kosntin   Broslev •   • Uman
Kresilev Letichev   Ladizhin   • Yekaterinoslav
Khmelnik   Monasterishtche   • Yelisavetgrod
Ulanov   Balte   • Savran   • Krivay Rog
Birzula • • Ananiev   Ukraine
Shvartz-Timeh ★   • Lyubashivka   • Melitopil
Korsn ●   Dnieper River
Bohslov ■   Odessa

Black Sea

Romania

now Germany. Over the centuries, much of this population migrated from the Rhine basin eastward, into present-day Poland, Russia, Ukraine, Belarus, Lithuania, Latvia, Czechia, Slovakia, Hungary, Romania, and Moldova. Today their descendants are known as *Ashkenazi Jews*, or *Ashkenazim*. Ashkenazi Jews have a long and complex history in Eastern Europe. Over the course of several centuries, through war, upheaval, and border changes, most of the Jews of Eastern Europe were eventually forced to live within a restricted geopolitical partition known as the Pale of Settlement (hereafter "the Pale") within the Russian Empire.

Inside this circumscribed zone, some Jews settled in larger cities, while others, under the auspices of wealthy non-Jewish landowners, founded small market towns, generally known as *shtetls*. Even though the political, legal, and geographic limitations of the Pale restricted many facets of Jewish daily life, these same constraints opened the door to intricate and intimate relationships with the non-Jewish communities alongside them. These regular connections with adjacent cultures had a significant impact on both the Ashkenazim and their neighbors. In this contested zone of ethnic, religious, and cultural confluence, Jewish, Slavic, and German traditions met, colliding or melding.[9]

Why is this significant and what does it have to do with folk medicine?

As more than one scholar has pointed out, the realm of health and healing, despite all the imposed limitations, had few or no boundaries in the Pale. Jews and non-Jews, whose lives intersected every day, borrowed freely from each other where health and healing matters were concerned:

> There is no field of science in which cooperation between Jews and non-Jews took place to a greater extent than in medicine. In spite of all the social, political, and religious restrictions—as far as Christian Europe is concerned—in cases of illness non-Jews sought remedies from Jews and Jews asked non-Jews for help. This applies to all classes of the population and to all centuries. Medicine alone did not respect any boundary.[10]

It should also be stressed just how important healing was to people over the centuries across the Pale, given the association of healing powers with Jewish religious authority: "Medicine's high value can be gauged by the remarkable number of famous rabbis [throughout their centuries in the Pale] who were themselves physicians."[11]

PIKUACH NEFESH

Some people might question the materials relied upon in Ashkenazi folk remedies that may not appear to conform to laws of purity. But Jewish doctrine has long held the view that the Jewish people must obey the commandment "therefore choose life" as a guiding principle.[12] Rabbis, as representatives of the religious establishment and often themselves healers, have always known how to resolve apparent religious contradictions by invoking the phrase *pikuach nefesh,* "saving a life." This principle in Jewish law affirms the necessity of preserving human life and overrides virtually any other religious considerations.[13]

Despite the attention that has been lavished on the world of religion and health, there is a wall that looms over this field, thwarting herbal researchers. Throughout the literature it's a given that Jews and non-Jews in the Pale shared healing knowledge with one another; in this selfsame body of literature, however, what goes undiscussed is the most important ingredient of the folk healer's craft: the medicinal plants themselves. Therefore, in order to rediscover exactly which herbs were known and employed by Eastern Europe's Jewish folk practitioners right up until the Second World War, we'll have to follow a long and exceptionally faint trail left by the elusive folk healers themselves.

Early Ashkenazi Healers in the Pale

In the Pale, many towns populated by Ashkenazim stretched along the trade routes that connected Eastern Europe to the larger world. Over the centuries, traveling merchants and traders who traversed these lands carried with them not only merchandise but news, information, and ideas from far-off lands. By the Middle Ages, the medicinal works of the ancient Greek writers such as Hippocrates, Galen, and Dioscorides had been translated into Latin and Arabic, making them accessible to broader audiences throughout Europe. These classical texts described plants and other natural substances and their efficacy in treating illness. Literate Jewish and non-Jewish healers alike drew from these sources for their work with plant medicine. The impression these works made on Jews practicing medicine in the Middle Ages can be seen in the reception of the writings of Moses Maimonides, a Sephardic physician, polymath, and philosopher who flourished in twelfth-century North Africa; his works influenced Jewish healers for many centuries.

In the Pale, from the earliest times, and even into the early twentieth century, causes of illness were understood differently than they are today. Contemporary medicine has shown that the symptoms of a cold, such as fever, are evidence of the body's immune system fighting off an invading pathogen, such as a virus. By contrast, healers in premodern Eastern Europe would have posited that a supernatural force, such as a demon, had caused the illness.

Of all the known supernatural forces, "the evil eye" made Jews of the Pale particularly wary.* Belief in the evil eye is an ancient concept, and while it's not specific to the Jews, mention of it is found in biblical writings. Those who feared the evil eye were convinced it was a curse cast upon the victim, motivated by envy or other malicious feelings. Often innocents such as children or animals were targets of the evil eye. The problems brought on by the evil eye could be almost anything: nausea, chest pains, headaches, weakness, or fear paralysis, to name a few. Curing the evil eye kept many folk healers busy in the Pale. As authorities in exorcising malevolent forces, experts were sought out both to cure illness and, for prophylaxis, to ward off potential harm.

THE BA'ALEI SHEM

So far we've only spoken about healers in general, but a variety of Jewish and non-Jewish folk medicine practitioners and healers flourished in the Pale for centuries: alchemists, pharmacists, shamans, and physicians all practiced variations of local folk medicine.[14] Foremost among the healers of many Eastern European Jewish communities were itinerant Kabbalists, or *ba'alei shem*, men who traveled widely, dispensing charms or incantations, amulets, and herbal remedies to combat the evil eye and other diseases for anyone in need of their expertise.

The ba'alei shem, "masters of the name (of God)," were a prominent feature of the Pale as both religious leaders and healers. The singular title *ba'al shem* signifies its bearer's ability to manipulate holy names, including those of God and angels, along with the names of Satan and malevolent spirits, in order to conjure desired results. The ba'al shem, as a cultural universal, served largely the same role or function as the shaman or "medicine man" in traditional societies the world over, mediating between the profane and the sacred, as an interceder between the living and the dead. Ba'alei shem were syncretic healers: relying upon the Kabbalah (writings of the Jewish mystical traditions) for guidance, and dispensing remedies both magico-religious and herbal, including amulets,

---

* If the term *kinnaherra* is familiar to you, it's a charm against the evil eye, from the Yiddish *ken ein hoyre* ("no evil eye").

traditional plant knowledge, and phamacopeia of the era to heal the individual and honor the Jewish mandate of *tikkun olam*, "repair the world."[15]

Their eclectic approach to healing made the ba'alei shem widely sought out by both poor shtetl dwellers and elites, whether gentile or Jew. These healers were extremely versatile, promising to restore vitality and fertility, cure disorders, particularly sexual disorders, and protect against sickness, misfortune, or the evil eye.[16] Ba'alei shem were also equipped with psychic powers of prognostication, fortune-telling, dream interpretation, and exorcism.[17]

Because Ashkenazim had for centuries shared with their non-Jewish neighbors a range of supernatural beliefs and practices, particularly with respect to the afterlife, the ba'alei shem were often consulted for protection from potential supernatural threats. Many Jews believed that the empty spaces surrounding towns or villages were the domain of evil spirits, such as Lilith of biblical renown, who lay in wait to kidnap newborn boys. Dybbuks, improperly buried persons (literally, "cleaving spirits"), might also assault the unsuspecting as they made their way to or from town. Most people believed these phantoms were dangerous, so safeguarding against potential attacks on anyone who might find themselves in potential disaster zones was essential.[18] To counteract a possible attack, the ba'al shem would create personalized amulets, incantations, and herbal remedies. As itinerant healers, they were sought out for a panoply of ailments and served as magicians, hypnotists, therapists, pediatricians, urologists, obstetricians, psychiatrists, homeopaths, parapsychologists, and family practitioners.[19]

Like their non-Jewish neighbors (i.e., later than their counterparts in western Europe), the ba'alei shem also eventually learned the mystical teachings of the physician and alchemist Paracelsus and incorporated them into their own healing methods.[20] Like other shamanic healers, the ba'alei shem interceded into the spirit world, but with a particular Jewish emphasis rooted in the Kabbalah with its reliance on Jewish ritual and symbolic magic.[21] A prescription for protection often included a handwritten personalized amulet, guaranteed to perform a wide range of functions. Each of these talismans was unique and had to incorporate four mandatory elements: the names of God and angels, relevant biblical passages or phrases attesting to God's healing power, a meticulous detailing of the object's various functions, and the name of the person it was meant for, along with their mother's name.[22]

In addition to their use of biblical sources for creating protective amulets, ba'alei shem also consulted special remedy books (generally referred to as *segulot*, "cures," and *refu'ot*, "remedies"). These resources were an integral part of Ashkenazi medicine from the Middle Ages onward and were consulted by Jewish folk healers right up until the Second World War.

THE REMEDY BOOKS

Besides their knowledge of religious history, religious law, and local oral traditions, the ba'alei shem relied heavily on the available medical literature. Their primary resources were the *segulot ve-refu'ot* remedy books, which circulated in both manuscript and print.[23] Remedy books came in a number of forms. There were "practical Kabbalah" guidebooks that borrowed liberally from popular Eastern European folk medicine beliefs and acquainted the Jewish reader with elements of Slavic superstitions, popular medicine, and healing practices.[24] Hebrew and Yiddish translations of works by western European physicians also served as remedy books.[25] While many remedy books were attributed to notable Jewish physicians or ba'alei shem, anonymous volumes were just as common, which suggests the intriguing possibility that some may have been written by women. The *Sefer ha-toladot*, which focuses exclusively on midwifery, is one lacking attribution.[26]

In the eighteenth century the Żółkiew press—at the time the only Jewish printing press in the Kingdom of Poland—mainly published books on practical Kabbalah.[27] These collections of recipes for an assortment of herbal remedies, charms, and amulets circulated throughout Ashkenazi communities for generations, but the introduction of publishing expanded their distribution and use greatly.[28] Because the Żółkiew remedy books incorporated so many Slavic popular medicine and folk beliefs, their content was quite distinct from many other publications in this genre, especially those emerging from Jewish communities in Italy, Germany, and the Netherlands.[29]

Most practical Kabbalahs were pocket-sized or slightly larger (duodecimo or octavo) and generally less than 150 pages. They usually contained an index of the most common diseases along with their corresponding healing remedies. For any given ailment, such a handbook might recommend a charm (such as the recitation of a specific psalm) coupled with an herbal concoction. To help Ashkenazi readers with the remedies, the authors would filter concepts and terms from Latin, German, Polish, and so on into colloquial Yiddish.[30]

Ba'alei shem, to best market their personalized services, wrote their remedy books to attract as wide an audience as possible. One remedy book, *Toldot Adam* by Yoel Ba'al Shem (also known as Yo'el Heilperin), enjoyed such enormous commercial success that its author boasted there was no town in Poland that did not have a copy.[31]

Some Herbs mentioned in the Early Remedy Books

Hillel Ba'al Shem, a well-known eighteenth-century practical kabbalist who traveled many of the regions of the Pale, in his Hebrew-language *Sefer ha-Heshek* relied on Polish and East Slavic dialect terminology—*plaster* (plaster), *kwarta* (quart), *wanna* (bath), *syrop* (syrup), *funt* (pound), *belladonna* (belladonna), *walerjana* (valerian), *majewij barszcz* (May borscht), *krapiwa* (nettles), *gorczyca* (mustard), *woronii koren* (raven root), *pijawki* (leeches).[32]

Yoel Ba'al Shem, who was active in Zamość (present-day Poland) in the late seventeenth to early eighteenth centuries, in his recipes used Slavic terms such as *tsybulia* (onion), *ognennaia kost* (fire-bone [elderberry?] seeds), *ruta* (rue), *malwa* (mallow), *smetana* (sour cream), *petrushka* (parsley), and "Slavic" herbs as well as medical terms (elixirs, balsams, plasters) common in the standard scientific language of the time.[33]

Along with practical Kabbalahs, the other significant genre of remedy books widely used by the ba'alei shem were the translated works of prominent European physicians of the era. The great international bestseller from the late eighteenth century into the nineteenth century was French Swiss physician Samuel-Auguste Tissot's *Avis au peuple sur sa santé*, "Advice to the People in General, with Regard to Their Health." Tissot's work went through many editions in a number of translations, eventually making its way into both Hebrew and Yiddish versions for the use of Ashkenazi healers in the Pale. Herbal products recommended by Tissot (all common in the general European *materia medica* of the time) in the Yiddish and Hebrew (abridged) translations include elderflower, silverweed, rose, purslane, lettuce, houseleek, vervain, herb Robert, crane's-bill, chervil, parsley, sage, rosemary, rue, mint, marjoram, tobacco, wormwood, ground oak, Carmelite water, and Hungary water.[34] Whether the remedy books were written by physicians whose work had been translated into Hebrew or Yiddish or were authored by the ba'alei shem themselves, this body of knowledge, which borrowed liberally from many sources both ancient and modern, left an indelible mark on medical praxis among Eastern European Jews, and many books were reprinted numerous times over several centuries.[35]

The European Enlightenment, the intellectual movement of the seventeenth and eighteenth centuries that emphasized the value of scientific reason over tradition, eventually affected the culture of Ashkenazi healers, whose practices were rooted in the age-old ways. And as the Enlightenment took hold in Eastern Europe, general communal trust in the traditional mystical ways of healers such as the ba'alei shem began to erode.

By the end of the eighteenth century, however, tsadikim (Hebrew, "the righteous"), the new leaders of the emergent Hasidic movement, which promoted a spiritual revival among Ashkenazim beginning in the eighteenth century, supplanted the ba'alei shem as community healers with paranormal powers; and the trained physician, along with a new profession, the feldsher, displaced them as community healers with medical or paramedical training.[36]

EARLY JEWISH PHYSICIANS

Alongside traditional healers and religious leaders, trained physicians also treated Ashkenazi Jews in the Pale. Prior to the seventeenth century, many Jewish physicians in Eastern Europe were formally trained in academies abroad, foremost among them at the famous medical school in Padua, Italy. Apart from practicing medicine for their livelihood, many Jewish physicians were also scholars, rabbis, philosophers, or poets. And while most Ashkenazi Jews were beset by persecutions, pogroms, forced conversions, and everyday restrictions and prejudice, trained physicians often attained high social standing in the communities where they lived. Significantly, these physicians often limited their practice to the upper classes rather than their co-religionists in the towns and villages. Many trained physicians considered themselves as too exalted to perform lowly tasks such as surgery, which they regarded as worthy only of their uneducated assistants.

Trained physicians in the early modern period (roughly 1600–1800) offered consultations or oversaw surgeries, but mostly they served as private doctors or university instructors.[37] Whatever advantages their formal education provided them socially or financially, the main contribution of early modern Jewish physicians toward the advancement of medicine was in their role as translators, bringing the writings of Islamic medicine (often via Hebrew) to a wider European audience.[38]

EARLY PHARMACIES

The pharmacy or apothecary has for centuries been the primary commercial source of medicaments, frequented by traditional healers and trained professionals alike: from the Middle Ages onward, pharmacies were where traditional and other healers acquired their secret ingredients, recipes, prescriptions, and jargon. Pharmacies sold not only preformulated medicines but also plants such as *Piper nigrum* (black pepper), *Cinnamomum* spp. (cinnamon), *Prunus dulcis* (almond), *Castanea sativa* (European chestnut), and *Laurus nobilis* (bay laurel) leaves, various roots, wax candles, and incense.[39]

Pharmacies served as meeting places for the ba'alei shem and other healers, where they could pursue their interests and trade stories and information regarding their arts.[40] In Poland the pharmacist was known as an *aptekarz, alchemik,* or *chemik,* and aside from supplying ingredients, pharmacists also relied on their own collections of books and manuscripts for recipes and instructions for concocting medicines. Apothecary libraries in all communities often collected not only classical medical tracts such as those of Hippocrates, Galen, Avicenna, and Dioscorides but also pharmaceutical and perfumers' manuals, along with the writings from the alchemical tradition. Among the most important alchemical works were those of Paracelsus and his disciples, whose thinking focused on the combined curative powers of magical belief and natural medicine.[41]

In the Pale, healers of different faiths and communities (Jewish, Russian, Polish, etc.) shared a trust in natural medical and alchemical remedies. Jewish Kabbalists, Polish paramedics, and private physicians of the Russian court were all engaged in the procurement and application of medicinal herbs. The inventories of commercial pharmacies in the larger towns of eighteenth-century Poland were made up of the same array of herbal concoctions relied upon by the ba'alei shem in the shtetl.[42] Jewish healers have left behind copious written evidence, such as handwritten prescriptions declaring *timtza be-apotek*: "You will find it in the pharmacy." These confident assertions indicate that the ba'alei shem were intimately familiar with the commercial and secular world of the pharmacy and its wares, the key resource for the unique elements necessary for formulating their healing remedies.[43]

EARLY JEWISH FELDSHERS

As mentioned previously, early modern Europe witnessed the expansion of a new paramedical profession, the feldsher. Paramedics were an integral part of the European medical landscape as far back as the Middle Ages. The complex history of the feldsher is tied to advances in both military technology and anatomical knowledge. In very general terms, feldshers were the military ("company") barber-surgeons, as opposed to the civilian barber-surgeons (known in Poland as *cyrulicy*) who practiced alongside doctors and traditional healers throughout Europe.[44] Cyruliks were trained in shaving and bathing (i.e., barbering) as well as setting fractures, bloodletting, treating wounds, and so on (i.e., surgery). The cyrulik's trade was often passed down within families, father to son, and many remedies were closely guarded secrets used over generations.

Attaching the barber-surgeon to armed forces to treat battlefield wounds and other afflictions common to military campaigns is what led to the rise of the feldsher, a word derived from the German *Feldscherer* (literally, "field-shearer"). The earliest feldshers specialized in the barber's trade, shaving soldiers and cutting their hair, but over time, as warfare and medical knowledge evolved, their duties became more complex, eventually including tasks such as setting bones, administering medications, cupping, bloodletting, surgery, and amputations. Ultimately the feldsher supplanted the civilian cyrulik, as the rise of large standing armies along with near-constant warfare created an ongoing supply of battled-tested, experienced paramedics throughout Europe.

While we will likely never know the first Ashkenazi Jew to serve as a paramedic, the historical record suggests that he may have served in Swiss mercenary forces as early as the thirteenth century. The documentation indicates that many Jews were community physicians tasked with combating epidemics. Given their representation in the medical trades, Jewish conscripts likely would have entered Swiss military service as feldshers.[45]

When the position of *Feldscherer* was created in the Austrian army, the feldsher (drawn from the ranks of the civilian cyruliks) made his official debut in Eastern Europe. By the early seventeenth century it was obligatory for every company in the imperial army to employ a feldsher.[46] It's almost a certainty that the army of King Jan Sobieski of Poland, legendary for his lifting the Ottoman siege of Vienna in 1683, included Ashkenazi feldshers: Sobieski's attitude toward Jews was extremely liberal, and while on the throne he granted the Ashkenazi communities of the Commonwealth many privileges and exemptions.[47]

In addition to working as battlefield surgeons—amputating limbs, affixing leeches, and stitching up lacerations—feldshers were responsible for administering medications and were expected to be knowledgeable about herbal treatments. Per a journal entry written by a late seventeenth-century feldsher who participated in Sobieski's campaign:

> *[Hospital] fumigation is carried out with juniper, wormwood, and even orange peel. The patients are treated with purgatives, emetics and perspirators. They do not spare the blood-letting and cupping glasses. They also heal with brandy, though it's difficult to get.*[48]

Herbal fumigants were a widespread treatment in Ashkenazi Jewish communities well into the twentieth century. In his memoirs, the Polish Jew Yuri Suhl (born in 1908 in Podhajce, present-day Pidhaitsi, Ukraine) recalled the room where his mother lay dying. With a good deal of effort, his father was able to buy an orange, a scarce commodity in those days. The patient was given the fruit to eat, and the precious rind was cut up and placed around the sickroom, the traditional method, according to the author, for clearing the contaminated air in the room of the infirm.[49]

Other early modern feldshers' natural healing remedies also continued to be used for centuries. The same seventeenth-century feldsher's journal notes the treatment for a gunshot wound:

> *On November 11, the feldsher applied herbal concoctions and ointment compresses . . . plasters of bread mixed with saliva and cobwebs to prevent*

gangrene and . . . when squadrons began to complain about frostbite . . .
ointments prepared from herbs that were excellent for prevention of the con-
dition were applied.[50]

Another twentieth-century Polish Jewish memoir, this from Apt (present-day
Opatów, Poland), attests to the persistence of this practice: the author reminisces
how, as a boy, he and his friends would use spiderwebs to bandage any cuts and
wounds they had suffered during a day's adventures.[51]

Nowhere in Eastern Europe was the feldsher as deeply integrated into
medical care as in Russia. Introduced into the Russian military in the seventeenth century, the feldsher, owing to a dearth of trained physicians and the
great size of the tsarist army, was a crucial component in medical service
in the Russian and later Soviet armies well into the twentieth century.[52] A
significant part of this expansion was precipitated by the late eighteenth-
century partitions of Poland and Russia's acquisition of much of its territory.
After 1795 most Ashkenazi Jews became Russian subjects, including any
feldshers who had served in the former Polish army and, with compulsory
conscription, would have subsequently continued their military service under
the Russian flag.[53]

The Russian government's treatment of its Jewish population was mutable.
During the partitions of Poland, in order to assimilate her new subjects into
the Russian Empire, Catherine the Great granted Jewish merchants permission to live and trade in the newly acquired towns in the districts of Mogilev
and Polotsk. Jews were also granted similar permissions in formerly Ottoman
regions conquered in 1793. These grants, however, were geographically fixed
into the notorious confines of the Pale of Settlement, which had been drawn up in
1791. These were the boundaries that restricted the movements and activities of
Russia's Ashkenazi Jews, and it was these discriminatory borders that persisted
for more than a century, right up to the First World War.

Under these complex circumstances, Ashkenazi feldshers throughout the new
jurisdictions continued to practice their trade and adapt to the dictates of the era
as best they could. If they managed to survive long terms of compulsory military
service, which at times was twenty-five years, they often returned to rural areas
of the Pale, where there was generally little or no sanctioned medical care, in
order to earn a living.

Several specific factors distinguished the Pale's Ashkenazi feldshers from their non-Jewish counterparts. While all of Eastern Europe's feldshers would have undergone similar on-the-job training, Jewish feldshers observed customs that made their healing methods distinct from those of other feldshers.

One of these differences lay in the simple act of shaving. Throughout the Pale, even as late as the twentieth century, shaving was prohibited for Jews. An Ashkenazi feldsher (or cyrulik), with a practice that mainly served his co-religionists, would not be expected to provide this service. Thus, unlike the Christian barber-surgeon, who might specialize in the former rather than the latter part of the hyphenated profession, his Jewish counterpart would have concentrated almost exclusively on the healing aspects of the profession rather than the tasks of grooming.[54]

Another difference lay in the Jewish feldsher's community standing. Because sanctioned medical care in Ashkenazi communities in the Pale by the nineteenth century was generally provided by feldshers rather than trained physicians (the restrictions that barred most Jews from attending Russian universities, along with the draft, played a large role in this), their social standing was rather high for a paraprofessional trade. Feldshers were considered "folk physicians" by their communities, and Ashkenazi Jews affectionately referred to their community feldshers as *rofe*, or *royfe*, Hebrew for "doctor." As they were so often "of the people," their down-to-earth reputation created a strong and trusting bond between feldshers and their communities. Assuming they were able to choose between a trained physician and a feldsher when seeking care, Jewish patients were far more likely to confide in the latter, particularly when discussing their reliance on traditional healing.[55] Because of their close and intimate ties to their communities (both as enforced through the restrictions of the Pale and the rooted hereditary lineage that shaped their practices), feldshers regularly interacted with other traditional folk healers, knew their remedies, and often made extensive use of that knowledge. As a result, the feldsher's medical repertoire was enriched by the variety of herbal and other traditional remedies they encountered.

A third difference that distinguished the Ashkenazi feldshers from their non-Jewish counterparts was their use of the remedy books, the *segulot ve-refu'ot* described earlier. These handbooks with their secret plant-based remedies were as important to the Jewish feldsher or cyrulik as they were for the *ba'alei shem*.

One of the most important works was the *Ma'aseh Toviyah* ("The Work of Tobias"), written by the physician Tobias ha-Kohen and first published in 1707, a cornerstone of the Ashkenazi feldsher desk reference for centuries. (Many manuscript copies and printings—from as late as 1908—are extant.)[56]

Feldshers of course also relied on secular European medical literature, such as Tissot. As these works went through the translation process, they were often reshaped to meet communal needs. One such book, Heinrich Felix Paulizky's *Anleitung für Bürger und Landleute* (1793) was translated into Hebrew (via Polish) as *Marpe le-Am*, and individual chapters were extracted, abridged, and republished (a pamphlet called *"Imrei Israel"* was a standard resource on convulsions). In its Hebrew rendering, *Marpe le-Am* was the key nineteenth-century medical text that incorporated Western medicine, traditional plant knowledge, and the specific religious requirements of the Jewish community; it was widely used by feldshers, physicians, and religious scholars alike.[57]

That the Ashkenazi feldsher relied on medical works with an explicitly religious focus indicates how strongly his approach to healing was directly influenced by Jewish religious sources such as the Talmud or other religious authorities (e.g., Maimonides). These sources generally contained detailed prescriptions for preventing disease by performing ablutions and exercises, the proper preparation of foods and beverages, and the benefit of massages, fresh air, and so on.

As for the Talmud as a medical resource, the majority of its healing prescriptions are based on well over a hundred plants and their derivatives, such as sage, rock soapwort (*Saponaria*), spinach, opium, and olive oil. Many of the Talmud's prescriptions, sometimes adapted but often unchanged, found their way into the feldshers' inventory as cures; baths in mineral water were advised for certain skin diseases, and purges using herbal enemas were also recommended.[58]

Feldsher medicines were mainly used to alleviate pain (opiata) or heal wounds through the application of different specialized ointments and plasters. The exact composition of many of these concoctions (reputed to have extraordinary curative properties) was often a jealously guarded secret. The most popular feldsher prescriptions in late eighteenth-century Russia for healing fresh wounds were the leaves of *Herba plantaginus* (*Plantago* spp.) or cabbage. Plantain has been recommended since ancient times for its curative powers. Tobias ha-Kohen in the

Ma'aseh Toviyah recommends it for digestive and related ailments; today's herbalists continue to utilize the plant for its ability to heal wounds and other afflictions. In the towns and villages of the Pale, *Plantago major* was one of the chief vulnerary herbs and was highly valued by traditional Ashkenazi healers. (See "Materia Medica": *Plantago major*, p. 177.) Feldshers also relied on common household ingredients when making plasters to apply to wounds: cotton.oil mixed with egg yolk, or wheat flour mixed with egg white or honey. For ointments the base was lard, bear grease, cotton oil, and laurel oil (*Oleum laurinum*).[59]

Given the religious proscription against pork, one might question the use of lard in ointments made by Jewish healers for Jewish patients, but it was not unusual for this ingredient to be cited as part of a prescription: for physical weakness, David (Tevle) Ashkenazi recorded in his book *Bet David* popular cures of the day that recommended the sick rub the soles of their feet with hog fat and drink boiled water with the juice of the gentian plant as a tonic.[60] This remedy is similar to one recorded in the early twentieth century in the town of Yelisavetgrod (present-day Kropyvnytskyi, Ukraine), where a folk healer, most likely a feldsher, gave to those suffering from colds an ointment made from dried nettle flowers mixed with lard, which was rubbed on the legs after a foot steam bath.[61] (See "Materia Medica": *Urtica urens*, p. 237.) Also relied upon by feldshers were "bear's ears" (uva ursi), taken as an infusion or dry powder for kidney ailments. Infusions of valerian leaves were drunk as a calming tonic, and valerian roots were swallowed as an emetic. Snakeweed ("Aristolochia clemat") was also a remedy for many ailments, and in fact, *Aristolochia clematitis* is one of the herbs employed in Ashkenazi folk medicine far into the twentieth century.[62] (See "Materia Medica": *Aristolochia clematitis*, p. 65.)

CHANGES BROUGHT BY THE ENLIGHTENMENT

The European Enlightenment inspired a specifically Jewish response: from the late eighteenth century, proponents of the *Haskalah* (Hebrew, "wisdom"), the Jewish Enlightenment, began to chisel away at age-old traditions, especially with regard to health and healing in the Pale. Physicians with Western academic training, together with health care reformers emerging from the nascent Jewish middle classes of Eastern Europe, attempted to reshape popular attitudes toward health care (along with reforms to education, culture, political and social engagement, etc.) as part of the new movement. By the end of the eighteenth century, as formal training and education became more accessible to Eastern European Jews, traditional healers—who lacked certifications and relied on the natural world for their remedies—attracted the scrutiny of the new Jewish scientific elites. The *maskilim,* proponents of the Haskalah, launched an offensive to reform the daily, intimate habits and customs of Jews throughout the Pale. Now traditional healers found themselves targeted by the new reformers.[63]

One of the most outspoken maskilim of the eighteenth century was the German-born Moses Marcuse, "the doctor of Königsberg." Today he's read mainly for his vivid description of Jewish life in Poland during this period, as recorded in his medical guide, *Ezer Israel. Ezer Israel* includes as an appendix (*Hanhagat ha-Refu'ot*), a remedy book derived from Tissot's *Avis au peuple sur sa santé* that cites many plants and herbal remedies well known throughout Europe at the time. In order to reach the Jews of Poland, his intended audience, whose healing and hygienic habits he believed were outdated and benighted, Marcuse deliberately rendered Tissot's work into Yiddish rather than Hebrew. In the introduction to *Ezer Israel* Marcuse accuses traditional Jewish healers not only of being complicit in this backwardness, but even responsible for all the ills of Eastern European Jewry:

> I had to write in Taytsh [a derogatory term for Yiddish, which Marcuse viewed
> as a corrupted form of his native German] because I wished to benefit many
> thousands of people with my book each year and to save them from such quacks
> and defectives as for instance, old women, bad midwives, exorcisors of the
> evil eye, bad epidemics, good air(?), evil and dirtied things, ignorant baalei
> shemot, and terribly wicked people; from pourers of wax [for magical pur-
> poses], from fortune-tellers who magically diagnose all diseases, from inept
> preachers who carry about remedies to sell for a good supper, for the sake
> of a small contribution and from worthless little "doctors" who have made
> themselves doctors, or have been made such by foolish old women.[64]

He continues his diatribe specifically targeting the feldsher:

> I have not yet mentioned our dear doctors or healers, who are called among us
> in Poland Rofe'im and Feldschers. I call them public, well-known specialists
> in killing, not Rofe'im.[65]

Marcuse's work did not garner the response he had hoped for, and his book disappeared into obscurity, only to be rediscovered in the twentieth century.[66]

It's tempting to imagine that Marcuse's disparaging opinions, expressed in "Taytsh," as he called Yiddish—a language he openly regarded with contempt—completely backfired, and rather than become a well-regarded standard medical resource, his book was instead relegated to the dustbin by the very healers he sought to reform.

The most rapid and far-reaching changes in Jewish medical care occurred in the half century before the outbreak of the First World War. The reorganization of the Russian public health care system, particularly the innovations of *zemstvo* medicine—a system of local governance that provided health care and other services to rural areas—greatly influenced the maskilim of the era. A steady stream of books and pamphlets of popular medical advice, written at first in Hebrew and later in Yiddish, were specifically produced for the benefit of Russian Jewry. Like Marcuse before them, these late nineteenth-century maskilim were determined to replace centuries-old customs with modern practices. The new advocates were convinced that health care reform was the essential necessary ingredient to better the living conditions of Jewish communities in the Pale.[67]

The maskilim, who championed the new "modern," "rational" health care practices as critical for the health of the people, perceived themselves as pitted against a well-entrenched enemy and even advocated against the harmful effects of a sedentary lifestyle, which meant denouncing the habits of the tradesman and yeshiva student.

The Jewish public health campaigns of the late nineteenth and early twentieth centuries painted their messages in tones more muted than earlier reformers such as Marcuse. Nevertheless, most writers continued the earlier attacks against all folk healers—that is, anyone other than university-trained physicians. They condemned the use of protective amulets and vilified traditional healers, labeling them "old women" and "sorceresses," among other belittling slurs. Even alternative medical systems such as homeopathy were pronounced illegitimate because they were seen as threats by the new medical establishment.

Just about every Haskalah work on health and hygiene published during this period included a section devoted to attacks on the "false healers." The difference between false and true healers was scientific education and official certification, which necessarily and automatically rendered all folk healers ille-gitimate precisely because they were outside the recognized scientific establish-ment. Only the physician, educated and academically trained, versed in the latest research, was regarded as the authority on health and healing. When confronted with cases where folk healers appeared to have cured illnesses, the maskilim physicians claimed the illnesses had simply disappeared on their own.

From the late eighteenth century, in an attempt to distance themselves from what they deemed the outdated ways, maskilim published their reform literature in Hebrew, the language championed by proponents of the Haskalah as another way to force Ashkenazim into the modern era. However, once it became obvi-ous the use of Hebrew was not tactically successful for achieving their goals (because most of their target population were not literate in Hebrew), these same advocates reprinted their offerings in Yiddish, the language spoken in everyday life in the Jewish communities of the Pale. It was only in the late nineteenth century, when the reformers made attempts to communicate in the vernacular, that they made significant inroads: the use of Yiddish in medical advice literature became a successful tool for raising mass awareness.[68]

Having cleared this communication hurdle, the maskilim doubled down on their reform campaign, taking advantage of a raging cholera epidemic that swept Russia in the 1890s. Pamphlets published at the time offered information and instructions for treating the disease while simultaneously warning Jews against all folk healers in the authoritative tone of medical science. From then, Yiddish-language public health pamphlets became a cornerstone of medical advice literature. Even popu-lar writers of the day, such as I. L. Peretz, were engaged in this work, adding yet another layer of populist authority via their celebrity endorsements.[69]

Women in particular were targeted because they were more open to discuss-ing such issues as contraception, sex education for adolescents, school hygiene, venereal disease, and their own health. But these campaigns were not univer-sally successful, despite lasting into the twentieth century. One memoirist recalls ordering for his wife a book, *What Every Young Mother Ought to Know*. The author admitted his spouse wasn't impressed by its advice:

> *She did not want to follow altogether the suggestions contained in the book.*
> *This may have been due to the difficulty of carrying into practice the instruc-*
> *tions given in the book, and it may also have been due to the fact that raising*

children in accordance with rules laid down in a book was then still unknown in those parts [of the Pale]. Be that as it may, I had to use a great deal of persuasion before she yielded.[70]

MODERN PHYSICIANS AND HOSPITALS

When the Russian government opened the doors of medical schools to Jews in the 1850s, Ashkenazim took advantage of this opportunity in significant numbers. It wasn't long before they were very much overrepresented (proportionally) in all branches of certified medicine: clinical medicine, pharmacology, nursing, midwifery, dentistry, and feldsher practice. While Jews, both men and women, were drawn to medicine for a variety of reasons, the groundwork for this entry into the professions was clearly laid by the assimilationist efforts of the maskilim.[71]

By the 1870s Jewish women were taking advantage of the (short-lived) Women's Medical Courses in Saint Petersburg, as well as official coursework in midwifery. Dentistry and, to a lesser extent, pharmacy science were predominantly female and Jewish fields, in large part because they were lower in prestige, pay, and privilege than clinical medicine.

Many Jewish physicians trained during this era—with the occasional exception of those from feldsher families—disassociated themselves from the Jewish masses while climbing the professional ladder, enhancing their social status by converting to Christianity, or joining the "assimilationists, declaring themselves Poles or Russians of Israelitic faith, changing their names to sound more Slavic, or refusing to speak Yiddish, instead speaking Polish or Russian only."[72]

As the number of Jewish physicians grew, the overwhelming majority chose private practice, intensifying the competition with the long-established feldshers. An increasingly powerful professional class of Jewish physicians and assimilationists railed against "feldsherism" in the name of social and medical progress, and they called for an abolition of the paramedics' trade.[73] As anyone can imagine, this further reinforced the animosity between adherents to the old ways and advocates for the new within the Jewish communities of the Pale. One story illustrates this contentious situation well:

Dr. Ezra who came to Eishyshok in the early 1880s . . . became a living symbol of the Haskalah in the shtetl . . . the clothes he wore, the fact that he sent his son to a Russian school in Vilna, his practice of bathing and swimming together with his wife rather than at sex segregated beaches, all these and many other departures from tradition acted as irritants to some of the balbatim *("bossy people").*[74]

Such airs had little effect on the townsfolk, who were perfectly aware of why many physicians had come to work in these rural communities: "He (Dr. Ezra) had come to Eishyshok because his medical license had been revoked, like other doctors who had had some sort of difficulty and had ended up in the shtetls."[75]

Despite the transformation of Ashkenazi Jewish society through the efforts of the maskilim and others, the Jewish physician in the Pale continued to share space in the medical landscape with the *royfe*, other Jewish healers, and healers of other faiths, including the Muslim Tatars and Christian Slavs (called *znakhari*, "those who know"). While their numbers declined over time, neither the folk healers nor their remedies were completely eradicated from the Pale. This can be ascertained through numerous sources, including interviews with elderly Ashkenazi immigrants conducted in Florida in the late 1970s. Many Ashkenazim (including a number of members of our own families), even after the Second World War, remained skeptical of (non-Jewish) physicians, maintaining their loyalties to the feldsher's care or a continuing reliance on herbal and magico-religious (e.g., amuletic) cures.[76]

Some of this embrace of traditional ways was due to the fact that in the Pale, with state resources often forbidden or unavailable to Jews, medical care was considered a matter of communal concern, and accordingly Ashkenazim had a longstanding, well-developed system of communal care. Where no hospitals existed, local Jews, out of charity, often hired physicians from the region to treat the poor. In almost every town, arrangements were such that local pharmacies would supply free or discounted medicine to the poor. Serving as crucial links in this network were the *bikur holim* ("visiting the sick") societies that helped provide necessary treatment and medication. Jewish charity also ran the *hekdesh*, the poor/sickhouses, which were notorious for their squalor. Most Jews accordingly were suspicious of hospitals and other such institutions as being dangerous to the patient—as a Yiddish newspaper pointedly expressed it in 1903, "When a Jew is taken to the hospital, he accounts it as if he is already being taken to *yene velt*" ("the other world").[77] With this in mind, it's easy to imagine why Ashkenazim may have preferred the care of traditional healers and their familiar remedies.

MODERN JEWISH FELDSHERS

Starting in the early nineteenth century, the Russian government established a number of schools in the Pale where feldshers could be certified, via examination, to practice as officially sanctioned civilian paramedics. But because of discriminatory hurdles to accessing education, most Ashkenazi feldshers did not bother with schooling; they simply chanced taking the examinations required for certification. While many Jewish feldshers may have lacked formal training, they would have acquired enough knowledge from their practice (whether military or civilian) or from studying the standard works—remedy books and popular works on health such as Tissot—to be able to pass the exams. In Congress (Russian-occupied) Poland, feldshers were required to display the traditional cyrulik's emblem of three copper plates on a rod outside their homes.[78]

Regardless of how they obtained licenses or certificates, by the late nineteenth century Jewish physicians, paramedics, and midwives were practicing in nearly every town in Congress Poland with a significant Jewish population; almost all towns with a Jewish population of at least twenty thousand (e.g., Kielce, Łódź, Lomza, Piotrków, Radom, and Warsaw) also possessed Jewish hospitals.[79] While smaller or less affluent communities lacked their own Jewish hospitals, or even resident physicians, practically every town had at least one feldsher. Most feldshers were retired from the Russian military and had moved to the countryside to continue earning their living through medical practice.[80] The feldsher was one of a core set of personages found in every shtetl:

> There was no Jewish community in Poland without its town fool. Just as a town needed its barber-surgeon, its bathhouse attendant-night watchman, and midwife, there had to be a meshugener, who belonged to everyone in common and whose welfare was the responsibility of the entire community.[81]

Note that the common denominator in this tongue-in-cheek account inadvertently underscores how seriously the obligation of communal care was honored by Jewish communities: every shtetl was assumed to have its health and hygiene needs taken care of by the feldsher, the midwife, and even the bathhouse attendant.

At the onset of the twentieth century, the importance of the feldsher for medical care was recognized throughout Russia; by 1905, forty-four civilian feldsher schools had been established, all with mandatory coursework in the use of herbal medicine among other healing modalities.[82] Despite this, unlicensed feldshers continued to practice, particularly in rural communities. For example, in Zarki (in the Kielce district of present-day Poland), there was no resident physician until the outbreak of the Second World War. Zarki did, however, have two paramedics, "Reb Aharon the Feldsher" and "Moshe Winter the barber."[83] The honorific "Reb" suggests the lingering association with piety and healing. As late as the 1940s, it was still common for the feldshers of Letichev (present-day Letychiv, Ukraine) to be affectionately addressed by local Jews as *royfe*.[84] Szczuczyn, in present-day Poland, was another shtetl that boasted several feldshers, in addition to a number of other health care practitioners.[85]

It may be difficult to calculate the precise number of Jewish feldshers who practiced in the former Pale between the two world wars, but the authors of *The Feldshers* offer this insight:

> In 1932, Radom (present-day Poland) had a population of almost 80,000, of whom thirty-two percent were Jews. [Among this population] there were fifteen Jewish feldshers and only four Christian feldshers. It can be inferred Jews clearly dominated the profession of feldsher, outnumbering non-Jews almost fourfold. It also reveals that despite the fact that no new candidates joined their ranks after 1921 [per the dissolution of the Pale and the laws that governed it], the Jewish feldshers were still represented in significant numbers.[86]

Why are these numbers significant? The Jewish feldsher, it may be recalled, was generally considered more trustworthy than the trained physician in many communities. Feldshers didn't need to obey the Haskalah populist dictum to "go among the people"—they were the people.[87] Their popularity among the Jewish masses was rooted in the customary communal respect Jews had for their own community healers. The persistence of this tradition—until well into the twentieth century—can be explained by the Jewish feldshers' emergence from and immersion within the most humble communities.[88]

But despite their ubiquity, these important folk healers are given short shrift in most histories of the Pale. Accounts such as this, from the illustrated reminiscences of a childhood in Apt (present-day Poland), recalling experiences from the period prior to the Second World War, are few:

> *Avrumele Sztruzer, another barber was also a feltsher (sic), a kind of para-*
> *medic . . . he had a library of medical books. People would go to the feltsher*
> *for minor ailments: colds, upset stomach, cuts and bruises, aches and pains.*
> *A feltsher could also treat ailments with bleeding and leeches or "pyafkes."*
> *I never saw leeches being used or bleeding but I vaguely remember over-*
> *hearing Luzer Klezmer talk about a cousin of his in Ozherov, a feltsher,*
> *who did bleeding. He apparently had a brass basin and scalpel for that*
> *purpose. What a feltsher could not treat himself he would refer to a medical*
> *doctor. . . . There was also Yudis, who had been an assistant nurse in the*
> *tsarist army [she may also have been a feldsher]; that qualified her as some*
> *sort of doctor.*[89]

While this aside may seem incidental, it does offhandedly acknowledge a woman practitioner whose existence at this late date (early twentieth century) was not unusual; however, little or nothing is documented of women's work, particularly women healers, at any time in the literature devoted to the Ashkenazi experience in the Pale. It seems probable that Yudis must have been a feldsher of sorts, retired from her military duties, to return to practice once again as a civilian feldsher in the small Jewish town of Apt, deep in the Polish countryside. These stories from Apt also mention an additional variation in the feldsher's trade, the bonesetter. But out of all these examples, the author can only recall the most sensational remedies, such as chicken droppings and saliva. He does, however, mention tobacco in passing, along with a mysterious bottle of "tincture," rare glimpses into the art of herbalism in the Pale.

Another early twentieth-century account describes a bout of food poisoning during a cholera outbreak in Horodok (in present-day Ukraine, near Lviv). The narrator faints, convinced that he is succumbing to the epidemic. He awakens to learn he's been cared for by the town rabbi and the local "surgeon apothecary," who assures him the danger has passed. This surgeon apothecary is most certainly a feldsher.[90] In a further mishap, this time in Kurenitz, another town in the Pale (present-day Kurenets, Belarus), a surgeon apothecary is summoned, and applies leeches, presumably for bloodletting, and then sprinkles his patient's injuries with a "powdered chalk" before bandaging.[91]

Meanwhile, in the Polish town of Eishyshok (present-day Eišiškės, Lithuania), a more contemporary researcher notes not only the presence of herbalism but also that of women healers among the community's members, who "did not use magic spells, but rather herbs and other folk remedies good for man as well as beast."[92] Eishyshok was yet another shtetl boasting two feldshers lacking academic training. These interwar practitioners were not only tolerated but eagerly sought out by both Jews and non-Jews alike for healing arts and techniques.[93] One of the remedies cited was to simply place raw potato slices on the patient's forehead to lower their fever, then replace with fresh pieces as the older slices warmed. This exact treatment was recounted several times in an informal survey I conducted in an Ashkenazi genealogy social media group in 2019.

MODERN PHARMACISTS

Alongside trained doctors and feldshers, who for many decades were invited from western Europe (England, Germany, France, Italy, etc.) by the tsars to practice in Russia, trained pharmacists were initially an imported profession.[94] In the early nineteenth century, in order to compete with pharmaceutical education in Germany and France, a number of professional schools were founded in Russia to train pharmacists. These new schools employed medical faculties and required students to pass highly technical pharmaceutical coursework in order to be awarded the official professional title of "Provizor."[95] By 1879 the Provizor examination had been further expanded so that students were required to demonstrate additional knowledge of science and scientific equipment.[96] In spite of the *numerus clausus* and other restrictions, a large percentage of pharmacy students, whose education included formulating plant medicines, were Ashkenazim.[97]

In addition to formulating and dispensing prescriptions, herbal and otherwise, entrepreneurial energy among pharmacists was an essential ingredient in the development of the Russian pharmaceutical industry. In line with the general economic and industrial expansion, pharmaceutical workshops, factories, and warehouses grew in number in the 1870s and 1880s. Ukraine, long a center for herb cultivation and export for the Russian Empire, became a key area for pharmaceutical production. Among the regions most known for herb cultivation for medicaments were the cities of Kharkov and Odessa, and Poltava province, all within the Pale of Settlement.[98]

Because it was against the law in some parts of the Russian Empire for Jews to dispense medication, those who were able to travel would venture further afield to buy their medicines in areas that permitted Jewish-run pharmacies. Nehmia der Feldsher of Eishyshok, for example, had two children who had left Poland to open their apothecaries elsewhere. Jews from Eishyshok had their choice of traveling north to his daughter Sonia's pharmacy in Vilna (present-day Vilnius, Lithuania), a mere forty-three miles away, or they could head east to his son Anshel's establishment in Ivenitz (present-day Ivianiec, Belarus), which was about twice as far.[99]

In spite of the fact that many Jewish pharmacists in interwar Poland could not dispense prescriptions, many drugstore owners did what they could to keep their customers, sometimes outmaneuvering the law whenever possible by continuing to fill prescriptions or by offering their own proprietary remedies, which were often secret formulations families had kept over generations. According to a contemporary author, some of these proprietary herbal formulas were still being produced almost a century later by descendants of the original Eishyshok inhabitants:

Hayya Sorele Lubetski's daughter for example still swore by her mother's cure for hepatitis: a drink made of ground up raspberry vines, dandelions and carrots, followed by a drink of a fresh chamomile infusion. Hayya Sorele also prescribed chamomile baths for yeast infections and infusions of chamomile for colds.[100]

In Eishyshok, the three Jewish drugstores were owned by Nahum Koppelman, Uri Katz, and Yitzhak Uri Katz. Among them they covered the necessities: the over-the-counter commercial medications that Jewish drugstores were legally permitted to sell and the familiar folk remedies that were always in stock. In addition they carried cupping glasses and leeches, urine compresses for use with animals, raw garlic to lower blood pressure, goosefat to prevent frostbite, blueberries to relieve diarrhea, stale bread or cobwebs for boils, and other health-related merchandise of the era.[101]

MEDICINE SHORTAGES, PLANT COLLECTION, AND FOLK KNOWLEDGE

By the revolutionary year of 1917, the First World War had strained the fabric of the Russian government, economy, and society. But the war also stimulated Russia's pharmaceutical industry. After the revolution, high prices and shortages of medicines and pharmaceutical supplies highlighted the challenges to the Soviet pharmaceutical industry.[102] To address shortages of materiel and resources, the Soviet government sponsored expeditions to collect known medicinal herbs throughout the country. (This was not unprecedented: two decades prior, Nicholas II had allocated 28,000 rubles to compile the first inventory of medicinal plants in Russia.[103]) Among the southwestern provinces of the former Pale, Kiev and Chernigov had the best-organized programs; more than thirty kinds of plants were collected in provinces home to large communities of Ashkenazim. Many members of the expeditions were schoolchildren and their teachers, who were recruited to gather plants such as the tropane alkaloid containing *Atropa belladonna* (belladonna) and the narcotic *Datura stramonium* (jimsonweed). *Valeriana officinalis* (valerian) was another medicinal plant gathered in large amounts.[104]

According to firsthand accounts of Ashkenazim from the town of Letichev in the Podolia region (in present-day Ukraine) who survived the Second World War:

> There was a vast array of herbs and spices used by local folk healers, doctors, and pharmacists of the region. Some Podolian herbs became so widely utilized that they were cultivated in a systematic manner, just like any other cash crop. It appears that herbal medicine was practiced not only by healers. Many people were aware of common herbs and their usages. Usually people learned how to recognize which botanicals had therapeutic properties since they were often asked as children to help the healers to search the fields for specific herbs.[105]

This recollection is further corroborated by a pamphlet written by a botany instructor from the Podolia region, titled "Cultivation of Medicinal Plants" (1916), advising potential growers on best practices.[106]

Between the wars, owing to scarcities of medications in the Soviet Union, a national campaign was launched to increase the quantity and diversity of medicinal plants. The campaign was carried out in the main by Soviet research institutions, botanical gardens, scientific academies, and universities, motivated in part to increase knowledge of medicinal herbs, classify and describe them, and replace expensive imported herbs with locally grown flora. Researchers assigned to these task forces conducted thorough and extensive investigations by observing and recording local communities' cultivation of and reliance on medicinal plants.[107]

Much of the research output from these expeditions remains relatively inaccessible, stored in post-Soviet archives, but some of this knowledge was disseminated in English. One study was focused on the medicinal herbs known by traditional healers in Ukraine and was carried out over a period of a dozen years between the wars. At a glance *Herbs Used in Ukrainian Folk Medicine* appears to detail the plants known exclusively to ethnic Ukrainian communities. On closer examination, however, the title proves misleading.

The study is presented as a clear-cut ethnobotanical examination of sorts; but no populations or communities are ever named. The only clues that describe the folk healers who were surveyed are the names of the towns where these informants lived. One brief passage detailing the study's interviewees reveals:

> It was important to know whether the population of the regions where the expedition planned to go had been settled there for a long time and whether or not [Soviet] collectivization had already been introduced. A stable, old, established population that has lived for many generations in the same place is more likely to have preserved ancient traditions and customs and mores, transmitted by word of mouth from generation to generation; this includes its knowledge of medicinal herbs . . . therefore the expeditions selected for their purposes the regions on the right bank of the Dnieper, where the population was well settled and where collectivization had only lately been introduced and thus had not yet disrupted the normal life of the villages.[108]

Even the most cursory examination uncovers some surprising facts. A remarkable number of the survey's inventoried towns that are located on the right bank (i.e., west) of the Dnieper River were squarely situated within the Pale; many of them had been settled by Jews in the eighteenth century or earlier. And, even more surprising, many of these towns and villages had maintained a majority Ashkenazi population, even into the late 1920s and '30s.

It's fascinating and exhilarating to contemplate that the very informants who relayed their herbal knowledge to the author of this study were most certainly the elusive Ashkenazi healers of the Pale of Settlement. And while the exact titles these informants held are not specified (unless in extremely generalized terms such as "villagers who were familiar with herbs"), it's possible to extrapolate from the medicinal plants reported in specific locations just who is speaking out from these few precious pages.

It's certain that the trusted feldsher, present in almost every community in the Pale for centuries, is well represented among the informants consulted for the study. As a folk healer, the feldsher would have been an obvious choice to consult, with indisputable expertise in folk herbal remedies traceable back through the centuries.

A second figure crucial to this story also emerges from the regions explored in *Herbs Used in Ukrainian Folk Medicine*: like the feldsher, the midwife also flourished in almost every community in Eastern Europe, but her role in history has never been well recorded. As an informant for a Soviet ethnobotanical study, the midwife has an undeniable presence, for a very large percentage of the medicinal herbs reported in the survey are dedicated to the support of gynecological health.

WOMEN HEALERS AND MIDWIVES

In his 2006 essay "An-Sky and the Ethnography of Jewish Women," Nathaniel Deutsch concedes that the Jewish women of Eastern Europe were rendered, in a variety of ways, virtually invisible. This often happened the moment they emerged into the world of the Pale, as it was common practice for baby girls to go unregistered at birth.[109] And, as noted earlier, religious and Haskalah elites alike had devoted little if any attention to the lives of women in their literary output—so little, in fact, that the population of the Pale might appear to have been made up predominantly of men. The following section attempts to reconcile this regrettable neglect with a brief focus on those women who were essential to the daily life of communities in almost every corner of the Pale: the Ashkenazi women healers who tended to the births, well-being, and deaths of Jews and other peoples of the region.

*Women have always been healers. They were the unlicensed doctors and anat-
omists of [Western] history. They were abortionists, nurses and counsellors.
They were pharmacists, cultivating healing herbs and exchanging the secrets
of their uses. They were midwives, travelling from home to home and village
to village. For centuries women were doctors without degrees, barred from
books and lectures, learning from each other, and passing on experience from
neighbor to neighbor and mother to daughter. They were called "wise women"
by the people, witches or charlatans by the authorities.*[110]

Along with feldshers, midwives are the traditional healers central to this story.
Despite only brief mentions in the Hebrew Bible and other Jewish canonical texts,
these women have been essential to the health of every community, in some form
or another, since humans have been born. Yet the midwife has been almost completely ignored in Ashkenazi literature regarding the Pale, except possibly for the
occasional diatribe, such as that of Marcuse in the late eighteenth century. These
women, who practiced tirelessly in the Pale and passed their knowledge from
mother to daughter for centuries, brought each new generation into the world. And
until official midwifery programs emerged in the Russian empire in the nineteenth
century, most managed to fly under the radar from literally time immemorial.

Out of the surfeit of male-dominated literature concerning life in the Pale, a
handful of deliberations and rabbinical responsa discussing the role of women
in health and healing can be gleaned. And from these often-harsh judgments,
glimpses of the humble midwife can be had. These stories are always matter-of-
factly told, neither embellished nor elaborated. Almost in spite of their lack of
detail, from these accounts the midwife stands out as an uncelebrated heroine,
bringing forth one generation after the other, but never once demanding even
the tiniest acknowledgment for her singular efforts.

The few accounts that surface in this literature are consistent across time and
geography. These women were required to take charge yet remain unassuming,
work without expecting praise or, in many cases, payment. In Apt, Poland, for
example, the midwife's presence during the most momentous of occasions is
only barely felt:

*As for babies, they were delivered at home by midwives. My friend Harshl recalls
there being two Jewish midwives: Itele and her daughter, Mrs. Warszawska. . . .
Everyone delivered at home unless there was a complication.*[111]

The much-celebrated eighteenth-century healer the Ba'al Shem Tov had his own significant midwife mentor, although her expertise was never credited:

Dor Zichroni, born in Medzhibozh, recalled a popular story about a woman who was having a difficult labor: "A man came to the Baal Shem Tov and he said, 'Rebbe, help me, my wife is in labor and she has been suffering more than a day now. She cannot have the baby. The midwife has sent me to you.' The Baal Shem Tov said: 'Bring your wife here.' When she came in the Baal Shem Tov gave her his big walking stick and told her to walk back and forth repeatedly. He then sent her back to the midwife, and she had the baby right away." It's possible that this remedy was passed down to the Baal Shem Tov from his mother, who was a midwife.[112]

At best, the midwife's role prevailed without comment. But if anything should go wrong with a delivery a midwife presided over, all complications were attributed to her. As such, it was almost reward enough just to be able to carry on the tradition: "The midwife was respected and loved but there was no status or *yikhus* (Hebrew, "prestige") involved."[113]

A recently translated memoir, originally published in Yiddish in 1910, touches on the life of the author's husband's grandmother, a much-respected community leader and midwife in the Pale. Because this woman practiced before formal education in midwifery became mandatory in Eastern Europe, her methods, captured in this recollection, are truly those of the traditional folk healer. And because she was a woman, her remedies had to have come from memory and were not drawn from a written source. Her expertise was available to both Jews and Christians alike.[114]

Two things about this memoir stand out as unusual. The first is its female perspective and author. The second is the inclusion of several specific medicinal plants the midwife employed in her work. Even such a scant account is unprecedented. Women's folk remedies were *never* written down (as opposed to the trove of information recorded in the remedy books that were consulted by male folk healers): their cures had always been transmitted by word of mouth, from one generation of midwife to the next, from time immemorial.

It's extremely fortunate that this author at the turn of the twentieth century inventories a fraction of her "grandmother-in-law's" traditional remedies that she recalled from having watched the woman practice her art. One of the remedies she preserved was a drink for chest pains and coughs, which was to be consumed for a whole month. The recipe, which calls for "oatmeal, cream butter and forty grams of candied sugars," seems completely at odds with what might be prescribed today for similar complaints. Other remedies prescribed by this midwife include a strong tea of sarsaparilla to be drunk over four weeks for the alleviation of rheumatic pain, blood stagnation, and headaches. Should the patient suffer foot problems, they were advised to soak their feet in baths of well-boiled green poplar leaves. The same midwife was also known to prescribe frequent baths to which were added a strong tea of "crushed hay crumbs, such as those found in a barn." Anyone who complained of vertigo was offered a dose of bloodletting as well.[115]

A large part of the Jewish midwife's responsibilities included infant health, and true to form, Wengeroff's grandmother-in-law was also remembered for treating children. According to her granddaughter-in-law, she administered baths with the addition of malt or the bark of young oaks to children afflicted with scrofula (a tuberculosis infection of the lymph nodes in the neck). This is identical to the remedy used by Poles of the same era for treating those weakened and debilitated by tuberculosis (See "Materia Medica": *Quercus robur*, p. 201). For bellyaches, the author writes, her midwife grandmother-in-law placed a mustard plaster on the stomach of afflicted toddlers.

This midwife's dedication is further acknowledged in a detailed description of a typical call for assistance in the wee hours. Because she had a large practice, she often got no rest at night. If someone knocked softly on her bedroom window and called her name, the old woman would pack up some medicines from the cabinet by her bed, dress quickly, and within minutes be ready to assist a woman in labor.

Midwives like the grandmother-in-law, who had been trained before the educational reforms of late nineteenth- and early twentieth-century Russia, continued to weave the ancient folk remedies into their healing practices. In another memoir from roughly the same period, a father-to-be has to make allowances for the old ways if he is to benefit from a midwife's expertise:

And presently we sent for the midwife . . . an elderly and experienced woman, who knew what was to be done in the case of a woman whose labor is very painful and prolonged. She at once gave orders for the doors of all closets to be opened wide and for the drawers of every bureau to be pulled out. I was greatly annoyed by this display of superstition but this was no time to talk philosophy to the women.[116]

Despite the dearth of information on these folk healers, the midwife's importance can be gauged by examining statistics regarding the development of medical training for women in Russia.[117]

As noted earlier, by the late nineteenth century all Russian midwives were required to be formally trained in all aspects of female health, including reproduction and infant care. In 1872 the Russian government began offering "Women's Medical Courses" as a four-year program at a number of institutions. After the first cohort graduated in 1876, the program was upgraded to a five-year commitment, equivalent to a university medical school degree. By that time, Jews comprised nearly one-quarter of all students in the program, and by 1879 one-third of students were Jews.[118] On the eve of the 1917 Russian Revolution, there were 6,000 trained midwives in the Russian Pale, all of whom were women, and nearly one-fifth of them were Ashkenazim.[119]

A short biography honoring one of Letichev's formally educated midwives, known as an *akusherke*, explains the requirements she had to fulfill in order to officially practice midwifery in the late nineteenth century. After traveling east to complete her courses at the Kharkov Midwife Institute, Sarah Gershenzwit Pulier, who had been born in Kamenets-Podolsky, returned to the Podolia region in the western part of Ukraine to settle in Letichev in the 1890s. There she raised a family and practiced her trade for over twenty years.[120]

By the second half of the nineteenth century and the decades following, an increasing percentage of women began appearing among the feldshers in Russian official records. This was directly due to the establishment of state schools for midwives in the Russian Empire. The graduates of these schools had the right to claim the double title of *fel'dsheritsa-akusherka* ("feldsher-midwife").[121] All of these graduates were expected to know the medical procedures of the era, including the application of many medicinal plant remedies.

But it's the personal stories left behind like so many forgotten breadcrumbs that reveal the extent of the midwife's herbal knowledge. Aside from heading to neighboring towns and villages to attend the bedsides of women in labor, some midwives traveled great distances and even pioneered new lands. In America, Ethel Krochock Bernstein's grandmother, Shana Gitl, was a spinner, herbalist, and midwife whose family had immigrated in 1890 from Kresilev (in present-day Ukraine, one of the towns visited by the interwar Soviet folk medicinal expeditions) to Grand Forks, North Dakota. Ethel recalled in an interview:

> My grandmother delivered me. She tied my umbilical cord and when the doctor arrived and saw what she had done, he said, "Very good, grandma." When medicine was needed for various ailments, my grandmother was taken to the drug store, and, incidentally she couldn't speak or understand English, was taken to a back room of the drug store where many herbs were in jars on shelves. . . . When she looked them over she pointed to this one and that one and took the herbs home and either ground or cooked them and made the medicine needed, and they always did the work expected of them.[122]

An archived photograph of Rosalie Gerut's grandmother, Raifka Fingerhut, notes she specialized as an herbalist in Novo Svenciani, Lithuania, before the Second World War.[123] Such accounts are significant because they provide further evidence of the consistent familiarity with medicinal herbs among Ashkenazi midwives and other folk healers throughout the Pale of Settlement. In addition, a number of Jewish genealogical websites list trades practiced by Jews of the Pale: for instance, Gesher Galicia (www.geshergalicia.org) inventories professions such as *Hebamme* (German, "midwife"), *fryzjer wojskowy* (Polish, "military barber"), and *cyrulik* (Polish, "surgeon").

A rare photograph taken in the Podolia region of Ukraine during the An-Sky expeditions just before the First World War shows a midwife with her "grandchildren" but tells only part of the woman's story. Its caption states:

> The models for midwives are the biblical Shiprah and Puah, who refused to fulfill the cruel order of the Pharaoh. Therefore, God "made them houses." (Exodus 1:15–21) In the folkloric tradition of Eastern European Jews, individuals kept life long ties with the midwife who delivered them and were considered her "grandchildren." The more "grandchildren" the midwife had, the larger was her share of the world to come.[124]

It's fascinating to read that these humble women were part of a child's world for their entire lives:

> The child will stand in a special relationship to the woman who attends his mother at his birth. He pays her visits and she participates in all the festivals and celebrations of his life. He gives her gifts especially when he is married

and he mourns at her funeral. She calls the children she delivers her "babies" and she in turn is known to all the community as "granny," [or] di Bobeh.[125]

Regardless of the midwife's low social status, it's clear Ashkenazim had a deep appreciation for these women healers and the crucial role they played in the communities of the Pale, as further demonstrated in the following excerpt:

Moshe's Mother Beila, the midwife of the "blessed hands" was respected as the busy "mother" of the majority of the town's children. She was always busy and whenever attending a delivery, had to prepare with her own hands all the necessary requirements; in many cases she had not been paid for her work at the birth of the previous child, but nevertheless would carry on quietly and efficiently. She continued to work until old age, being replaced by Edzia, Itshiale's wife. The respect the people had for Beila could be seen when she died and all the mothers lit candles at her deathbed and around the house. A candle was lit for every child she helped to bring into the world. Thus, there were thousands of candles. A sight that no one who saw would ever forget.[126]

Two things about Beila's story are, surprisingly, not unique. The first is the lack of importance placed on financial payment for the services rendered by a traditional healer. It seems evident that it was not remuneration that motivated most folk practitioners in their work because they were not typically paid for their services, consistent with the general ethos of all medical care in Russia over the centuries. The second demonstrates a now extinct rite of passage: the candle commemoration. This forgotten custom was observed in most Ashkenazi communities throughout the Pale and, fortunately, was recorded by an ethnographic expedition that took place around the turn of the twentieth century.

THE AN-SKY EXPEDITIONS

In an attempt to document the disappearing folk traditions of the Pale's Ashkenazim, the 1912–1914 An-Sky ethnographic expeditions began to collect their "tales, legends, sayings, spells, remedies and histories told . . . by men and women."[127] The bulk of the information gathered remains to this day somewhat inaccessible to researchers; however, a few exhibitions of recently rediscovered photographs, including those of the "grandmother" midwife mentioned previously, have been published within recent decades.[128] These publications add visual and anecdotal evidence that further elucidates the herbal and other folk cures that had persisted within Ashkenazi communities, right up until the Second World War.[129]

An-Sky, a pseudonym for the Russian-Jewish ethnographer, journalist, and playwright Shloyme Zanvl Rappoport, organized the first comprehensive ethnographic study of the Ashkenazim of the Pale. Influenced by similar ethnographic work conducted elsewhere in the Russian Empire and Eastern Europe, An-Sky planned two separate tours of the Pale; unfortunately, only the first came to fruition. (Interestingly, the interwar Soviet folk medicinal expeditions in Ukraine discussed earlier would visit many of the same towns on An-Sky's route, possibly retracing his steps.) The second half of his epic project was intended to gather information by means of an exhaustive questionnaire designed to elicit detailed descriptions of the customs and day-to-day activities of Eastern European Jews. Before the ambitious plan could be finished, the First World War erupted and the expedition was abandoned. But the questionnaire, while never used as intended, remains intact and functions as a historical document in its own right. With its extremely detailed enquiries, it illuminates many cultural practices that have never been explored, particularly with regard to women's lives.[130] A smattering of questions devoted to pregnancy and childbirth, the area in which men were almost entirely absent, exposes both the expected banalities but also details a few traditions now long lost.

Let's return for a moment to the memory of Beila of Zamość (present-day Poland), the midwife whose "grandchildren" were engaged in a candlelit procession at her funeral. The following entry taken directly from a translation of the An-Sky questionnaire makes clear to the reader that Beila's candlelit commemoration was only one instance of a much more widely practiced communal rite: "Is there a custom that when the midwife dies, all of the children whom she brought into the world accompany her funeral procession with candles in their hands?"[131]

While the questionnaire reveals many previously unknown day-to-day common practices of Ashkenazim, especially with regard to Jewish women in the Pale, a very unexpected pattern also takes shape: the cross-cultural parallels between Jewish women and their non-Jewish neighbors. Of particular significance are the areas of healing and exorcism. These connections once again confirm that Jews and non-Jews frequently interacted with one another, sharing the intimate knowledge inherent in traditional medicine.[132]

FORGOTTEN TRADITIONAL WOMEN HEALERS

In an unusual acknowledgment of women healers' varied experiences, *The Shtetl Book*—published forty years after the Second World War and contemporary with the achievements of the Women's Movement—begrudgingly gives readers a keyhole peep into yet another type of woman healer in the Pale. A short section entitled "Women at Work" mentions a few healing practitioners who stand out against a random list of feminine occupations: the "herb vendor," a syrup maker, a "medic who healed with leeches and other folk remedies" (whom we can now safely identify as a feldsher, and possibly also a midwife), and an "opshprekherin," a woman who gave advice and remedies to people convinced they had been cursed by the evil eye, an affliction cited in the Talmud that had to be cured before it caused further illness. Such a spare litany of occupations would seem to suggest that "Women at Work" did nothing worth elaborating; but with a little extra digging, we discover something much more intriguing.[133]

In addition to their previously noted revelations, the An-Sky expeditions confirmed that the opshprekherin had survived into the twentieth century.* The practice of the opshprekherin was rooted in the ancient belief in the evil eye. Mostly women, these healers were present in almost every town in the Pale and were sought for their expertise in times of crisis, during pregnancy, for toothache, a bad foot, an abscess, a "rose" (erysipelas skin infection caused by *Streptococcus* spp. bacteria), the bite of a mad dog, epilepsy, or any other maladies believed to have been caused by this curse. The opshprekherin never referred to written sources for her cures; hers was an oral tradition deeply shrouded in secrecy:

> *Pregnant women—especially when carrying their first child—often asked these older women for protection [for their baby from the evil eye]. People believed not only that the opshprekherin had the power to predict an unborn baby's gender but that they could in fact influence whether it would be a boy or a girl. Those old ladies had a supply of "proven" charms and spells for each occasion. They performed magic with knives, socks and combs; they poured wax and poached eggs and knew hundreds of ways to cure a patient.*[134]

---

*Most of the sources cited throughout do not mention this healer by her Yiddish title. It must be inferred from the expedition text that these are the same healers as those described in other sources since the specific details of their craft are identical.

In an informal survey I posted in a social media group while researching this project, many respondents, including one of my father's cousins, vividly remembered their childhood colds had been cured by the sock their mother had placed around their neck at bedtime. This practice may have its roots in the traditional healing services once rendered by the opshprekherin. Most of their remedies, however, they kept closely guarded.

> The old women were very careful not to divulge their secret spells and remedies to others; they even refused to tell members of their own family. They seem to have felt that if they revealed a spell or secret remedy to anybody else they would be giving up part of their powers and so would inevitably become weaker. Moreover, being guilty of a sort of treachery, they would themselves suffer some form of retribution if they ever used those spells or medicines again.[135]

Folk healers from adjacent Eastern European cultures also expressed similar reluctance when asked about their remedies. We will see later that this is another parallel Ashkenazi healers had with their neighboring equivalents.

More popular than the ba'al shem, the female opshprekherin also played a crucial role over a longer time period. These practitioners had already been well established as reliable folk healers at least as early as the 1700s and can be glimpsed within Marcuse's tirades of the eighteenth century: "I have already warned you in my book against ignorant ba'alei shem, Tatars (i.e., soothsayers), wax-pourers, exorcisers of the evil-eye."[136] Even modern writers, such as Abraham Rechtman, a member of the An-Sky expeditions, are withholding when describing the practices of the opshrekherin, whose methods, he wrote, included the wax ceremony. H. J. Zimmels in *Magicians, Theologians, and Doctors* also briefly mentions these "medicine women" who cured diseases with their expert recitation of charms, and in cases where the evil eye had to be exorcised, wax was poured during the ceremony.[137]

In yet another account of an opshprekherin at work, a poorly translated description regarding the wax ritual has misled readers for decades. The story can be found in "The Healer from Bilgoray," part of the classic collection *From a Ruined Garden*: "In cases where someone became paralyzed, Sore Mordkhe-Yoysef was sent for, she would pour wax over the person's head and point out reasons why he had become frightened."[138] This passage, though badly garbled, describes an opshprekherin performing a kind of exorcism. However, the translator omitted the most salient portions of the act and misinterpreted the meaning of several words, leaving the reader with the impression that a woman named Sore Mordkhe-Yoysef poured hot wax over someone's head and then told that person that this was the reason they had become frightened. The passage actually states that when the client was paralyzed or *"gekhapt"* ("caught"), Sore Mordkhe-Yoysef poured wax above their head to determine the signs (*"simunim"*) indicating the cause.[139]

Incredibly the traditional wax ceremony has survived into the twenty-first century. But today its practice in Eastern Europe is largely limited to Ukrainians. A contemporary anthropologist studying the wax ritual described it more accurately this way:

> *During the wax ceremony, a patient who comes to a healer for help is seated in a chair. A bowl is filled with cold water and a lump of wax is melted. The healer engages in conversation and asks the patient for his or her symptoms. An incantation is uttered and the wax is poured into the water over the head of the patient. The solidified wax is taken from the water and turned over and its shapes are interpreted. The ceremony is considered effective in curing fear sickness and numerous other maladies.[140]*

In the Pale when someone became "paralyzed" with fear, or had fear paralysis, they sought out help from those who specialized in removing such maladies. The opshprekherin, who frequently interacted with women healers from neighboring cultures, borrowed remedies from these women and in turn shared her recipes and charms with them.[141] But because opshprekherins no longer exist to describe their work, and because there are no known accounts dedicated to these women or their practices in the established literature concerning the Pale, we must rely on the descendants of those healers with whom the Ashkenazi medicine women would have had contact. In this way we are able to better appreciate these forgotten traditional Jewish healers from a not-so-distant past.

Some of the contemporary folk healers who continue to perform the wax ceremony are Canadian Ukrainians who originally emigrated from western regions of Ukraine, where they had lived in close contact with Ashkenazim in the heart of the Pale. Mostly women, they go by names that are varied and include *baba* (old woman), *baila* (murmurer), *chaklunka* (conjurer), *chudesnytsia* (wonder-worker), *potvornytsia* (seer), *sheptukha* (whisperer), *zolotarykha* (golden conjurer).[142]

In the province of Alberta, the wax ceremony is called *vylyvaty visk* or *strakh vylyvaty* and can be loosely translated into English as "pouring wax" or "pouring fear." The ceremony has elements of Christian as well as pre-Christian imagery and is always performed with an accompanying incantation of a ritual prayer. This form of folk medicine was widely practiced in Ukraine and was easily transplanted to Canada as it required materials that were common to both the old and new continents: a bowl, water, wax, and the incantation.

Those who continue to seek the expertise of these healers do so because they are bothered by a fear they would like to be cured of. Fear can manifest itself in many ways: as emotional or mental illness, dread, anxiety, or general unhappiness. Physical problems such as weak kidneys (resulting in bed-wetting among children), speech impediments such as stuttering, tremor and epilepsy, anxiety, insomnia, or general nervousness or tension are also thought to be symptoms caused by untreated fear. At times these contemporary healers are known to include various plant and animal ingredients to address such conditions.[143]

The Ukrainian wax treatment, typically applied over three separate sessions, has been considered generally successful and is known to further enhance the healer's reputation. Because of the religious nature of the remedy, it has been widely tolerated even by the church (whatever the denomination). A clergy person in Edmonton justified the practice by saying it was a conduit for the healing powers of God and therefore did not go against church beliefs or practices.[144]

Aside from the obvious parallels, several other interesting similarities should be noted. The justification given by the church official for tolerating the practice is very similar to those given by rabbis who invoke the rule of *pikuach nefesh* for practices that, under other circumstances, might be considered heretical. In addition the Canadian practitioners were often hesitant to speak about their work because they feared their healing abilities might be revoked by higher powers or turned against them by unknown forces. These evasions were shared by both the contemporary Ukrainian healers and the opshprekherins who were interviewed by the An-Sky expeditions a century earlier.[145]

Another parallel can be seen in the case of Ukrainian children who were afflicted with a fear or possibly being bewitched (*navrochuvaty*) by the evil eye (*uroky*) and therefore could be the beneficiary of the wax ceremony. Treatments for these conditions consisted either of "pouring off the fright" or throwing coals (*vuhlia shydaty*) to produce a cure, either of which was often successful.[146]

This concern that children might be the intended target of an evil eye was also well-known among the Ashkenazim of the Pale. In Apt, Poland, a writer recalled how his baby brother cried so inconsolably that their mother became convinced someone had given the infant the evil eye. She based her fear on the fact that he was a beautiful baby who often attracted envious glances. The mother sent her older son in the middle of the night to a neighbor, Reb Moyshe Yitskhek, who was known for his ability to exorcise the evil eye. The boy woke Reb Moyshe to explain how his brother would not stop crying and his mother's suspicion as to the cause. The old man asked for the boy's parents' names and the baby's name, as was the custom, and after he had gotten this information, turned to a corner, murmured an inaudible prayer, then told the boy to go home. By the time the child reached his house, his little brother had stopped crying and fallen asleep.[147]

These murmured prayers, or incantations, were considered a powerful part of an exorcism. Often kept secret and uttered inaudibly, the incantations heightened the mysterious aura of the healing process for both patients and healers who believed the ceremonies would be ineffective without the accompanying intonation. The recitation and its whispered quality are yet more parallels between the respective rituals of the Jews and their neighbors. Sources including Abraham Rechtman of the An-Sky expeditions have described the whispered quality of these recitations along with the atmosphere of mystery and divine otherworldliness such mutterings lent to the patient's cure.[148]

Opshprekherins in the Pale interviewed by the An-Sky teams were recorded reciting their charms, which they uttered in Yiddish or in the tongue of a neighboring culture. At times the charms could incorporate Christian words or beliefs. One medicine woman, Hinde di Tikern or Tukern ("woman administering ablutions to women"), who was recorded by Rechtman during the first An-Sky expedition, spoke to her interviewers in Ukrainian. Her whispered recitation was transliterated from the spoken Ukrainian to the Hebrew alphabet then later translated into and published in Yiddish. This is her charm, rendered here in English:

> *Evil eye, I exorcise you (cast you out), out of the neck, out of the forehead, out of the chest, out of the shoulders, out of the spine, out of the ankles, out of the*

fingers, out of the stomach, out of the back, out of the feet, out of the elbows, out of the knees, out of the whole body. Are you an evil eye, are you a pest, are you an annoyance, have you come by sight or by thought. Do you happen once, twice, or thrice? Did you come from far away, or from another time? Are you of the morning, are you of the evening? I cast you out . . . Did you come from the eye of a Prussian, of a Gypsy, of an Englishman, of a Jew? Or from a woman, or from a man. Or from a girl. Or from a boy. Or from a calf. I cast you out from bones, from blood, and from the whole body. You shall find no happiness there, you shall find no refuge there. You shall not feed on the white body. You shall not drink the red blood. You shall not break the yellow bones. I cast you out . . . send you far away, into the marshes, out onto the blue sea, into the stone fortress. There you shall find happiness, there you shall take refuge, there you shall feed on dust, and stones. Blessed be that desolation in the face of the lord, and of all the saints.[149]

Comparative readings of Ashkenazi incantations against those of adjacent communities show so much overlap that it's impossible to deny their similarities. The following is an English translation of a Ukrainian wax-pourer's recitation recorded in the late 1990s in Canada:

I am not blowing away dust, but fear. I am not blowing away dust but fear and sickness. I am not blowing away dust but fear, sickness, hatred, nerves, and the Evil Eye. To disappear and vanish from [name's] head, from [name's] heart, from [name's] viscera, from [name's] upper back, from [name's] lower back, from all joints. Do not drink red blood, dehydrate a white body, or strip a yellow bone. By the heart do not appear, do not make yourself a nest. Disappear and be gone in the name of good fortune, of health.[150]

In Eishyshok, as in other Jewish settlements in the Pale, the practice of folk medicine thrived for generations, coexisting with more modern medicine into the mid-twentieth century. And like in the rest of the Pale, the methods of healing ran the gamut of strictly magico-religious to mainly herbal and every combination in between. Incantations noted there included those spoken in Yiddish, Slavic dialects, and Tatar—many Ashkenazim considered the Tatars as the most adept of the folk healers.[151]

Consider this magic spell that was recited against toothaches in Hebrew and meant to be repeated three times:

Once as Job was walking on the road, he met the Angel of Death.

Said the Angel to Job: "Why are you so engrossed in pain?"

Job replied: "Because of my aching teeth." And the Angel said to him: "As the desert has no seashore, so the teeth of the son/daughter of So-and-so will ache no more and will be mighty as the Hebrew letter Shin. In the name of the bone, Amen Sellah."[152]

While a possible explanation for the mixing of languages and symbols may be due to cultural borrowing, it's difficult to figure out which direction these shared prayers came from. Some similarities are obvious, like the identification of the disease and the remedies, the litany of enumerating objects such as human body parts, the naming of those who might have caused the illnesses, other diseases, positive or negative numbers, and so on. These elements are represented in both Jewish and Slavic folk incantations.

Another magic spell used for toothaches in Eishyshok was spoken in Russian mixed with other dialects and addressed the three tsars: the tsar of the high skies, the tsar of the fertile lands, and the tsar of the distant seas. It was only to be recited at night when the moon was shining, conjuring the power inherent in a specific phase of the moon. It was possible in Eishyshok to hear magic spells for many ailments including snakebite, headache and stomach cramps, the evil eye, or a blanket spell to cover all discomforts.[153]

In many Eastern European cultures, wax was not the only substance accompanying the incantation and employed in folk healing traditions. Lead and solder as well have been documented as sacred vehicles for similar ceremonies. Along with wax, these substances all have a relatively low melting point and can be poured into cold water to solidify quickly and then be interpreted by a folk healer.

Intact raw eggs were another agent traditional practitioners used to sense illness in a person, as were "coals," fragments of charred wood that were cast on water to determine if a person's affliction was caused by the evil eye.[154] Coal, or charcoal, is mentioned in Jewish sources as an object capable of divination. Marcuse himself remarked on the use of embers, or charcoal, in a ritual ceremony conducted by folk healers of the period.[155] And over a century later, in the early twentieth century, traditional Jewish healers were still practicing this custom with the very same objects. In Biłgoraj, Poland, when someone became sick and could not afford a doctor, burning coals were tossed into a glass of hot water on their behalf. If the coals sank, it was a sure sign the evil eye was the cause of the malady. And once this was determined, as in the Apt story of the crying baby, a child would be sent to seek the healer, apprising them of the situation and supplying the name of the infirm and the name of the sick person's mother.[156]

In Eishyshok lead was used in place of wax to discover the reasons someone had become incapacitated by fear or moodiness, restlessness or depression. A lump of the metal was melted in a frying pan and, like the wax, poured into a bowl filled with water that was held over the invalid's head. Once the substance solidified, its shape was interpreted to find the source and cure for the affliction.[157]

The Biłgoraj opshprekherin also used burnt flax and a charm recitation to begin her ceremony to heal a case of erysipelas: "Black royz, into the field, into the field." Afterward she applied honey, today a well-known antibacterial, to the infection.[158] In some ways, the incantation can be viewed almost like religious theatrics necessary to help a patient psychologically triumph over their illness, while the true physical medicine, in this case the antibacterial honey, was hiding in plain sight.

Yet another memoirist recalls two folk healers in an Eastern European town who were known exorcists of the evil eye. One of these, an opshprekherin, employed a method curiously close to the *limpia* ceremony practiced by the shamans of the Americas. Golda, the preacher's wife, as learned as her husband, knew how to remove or cure an infection presumably caused by the evil eye. She would simultaneously whisper a charm to herself while gesturing around her patient's infection with an unbroken raw egg in each hand to remove the spell.[159]

The other town folk healer applied another combination of magical object and inaudible incantation to remove the evil eye:

> David the carter, who delivered flour from the mills to the shops . . . used to neutralize the evil eye by means of small bones from a human skeleton. To this day it remains a mystery how he came by those small bones. If anyone's face swelled, in other words, if his cheeks swelled up due to an infected tooth, as it is called, or if he suffered from a sore throat, he would go to David the carter. He would take hold of those small bones and circle the swelling with them, all the while whispering incantations to himself. And the patient was convinced that, if not at once, then the next day or the following week or so, the swelling

would disappear. There was no doubt in the minds of the town's inhabitants that the swelling was caused by the evil eye.[160]

To quell any accusations of heresy against healers for reciting the possibly offensive, one religious authority granted them permission to continue their work because only the sounds of the words recited and not their meanings had a healing effect. Another declared that incantations were an illusion whose healing purpose was to bring tranquility to the mind of the patient and as such posed no threat. Yet another authority—who worried the potential sharing of ideas between adherents of different religions or the possibility of a rabbi being asked by his non-Jewish neighbors to devise a personal amulet or even to pray for them—finally consoled himself by acknowledging that many of these folk medicine practices were widespread and long in use, some so ancient their origins could not even be traced. He eventually ruled that any potentially questionable remedies were absolved by the mitzvah of "saving a life" or *pikuach nefesh*: "He who acts quickly is praiseworthy. He who refrains from doing so is regarded as if he had shed blood."[161]

THE WET NURSE

While not healers in the strictest sense of the word, wet nurses offer another possible clue as to the close connections between Ashkenazim and neighboring cultures when it concerned the health of community members:

> *The wet nurse, like the midwife, has a special and lasting relationship to the child. Her own child is the "milk sibling" of the one she has nursed. Although it is better to have a Jewish nurse, in many places, even the Orthodox employ a peasant woman if they need and can afford the luxury of a wet nurse. Undoubtedly this practice has contributed to the mingling of Jewish and non-Jewish superstitions and magic practices so that it is often difficult to tell which group has borrowed from the other.*[162]

In Apt, we find a more personal story concerning this close relationship:

> *Jadwiga was my mother's wet nurse. Jadwiga always managed to have a child at the same time as my grandmother did; this was how she was able to nurse six of Grandmother's children for her.*[163]

In later years the same family took Jadwiga in when she had nowhere else to go. When she became sick, they saw to it that she was properly taken care of and had a respectful burial when she passed away.[164]

LAMENTERS AND MOURNERS

Even though medicinal plants were not part of her protocol, the professional mourner also played a significant role in the healing of Ashkenazi communities of the Pale and deserves acknowledgement in this story. Women mourners can be traced back to biblical times. An-Sky's thorough survey describes for us (question number 1719) the important role the lamenters played in the community. Had the second expedition taken place, it would have required audible recordings of any versions of their songs.[165]

In a cemetery in the town of Nemirov (present-day Nemyriv, Ukraine), a trio of these lamenters appears in a photograph taken by the first An-Sky expedition in 1912.[166] And in the town of Zabludove (present-day Zabłudów, Poland), Esther-Khaye, a professional mourner, is remembered in this way:

> Women stand waiting for her as if she were the greatest celebrity. Not only the people of Zabludove, but even strangers who come to visit their ances- tors' graves know her already. Who doesn't know that with her "saying" she can move a stone from a pit? No one can remain indifferent to her "saying," not even menfolk. . . . The way to the graveyard is not far from town, and as Esther-Khaye enters, she feels at home, among people she knows. "Good morning, God," she begins in a tragic melody. "Your servant Esther-Khaye has come." And approaching the grave, she looks over at the woman on whose behalf she is supplicating, and words begin to pour out of her mouth as if from a spring.[167]

Mourning women were known by many names—*baklogerins, zogerkes, klogvaybers, beterkes, klogmuters, platshkes*—and were a feature in most Ash-kenazi communities.[168]

In one story, a narrator acknowledges the professional mourner is not only called upon for funerals but also often sought out to ask one's ancestors to help their living relatives with day-to-day problems. Difficult childbirths or dan-gerous illnesses were just two of many possible reasons for their intercession.

Carrying candles, wicks, and other necessary supplies, a mourner approached the grave of her patron's relatives and called out the name of the deceased, and with her fist she struck the gravestone three times. Because the ancestors were already in the afterworld and therefore closer to an entity who might be able to assist with any given worrisome situation, the prayers the mourners recited were believed to produce a more positive result than anything the still-living sinners of the world could enunciate:

> How can you be still when your daughter is in need of health and livelihood? Exert yourself for her sake, pray to the Lord of the Universe, after all you're somewhat closer to Him than we sinners, be an intercessor on behalf of her and all of Israel and let us say, Amen.[169]

In Apt the women mourners were remembered in a more haunting way. There they were called *di platshkes* (from the Polish word *płakać*, "to cry"). Families would hire them when a relative was on their deathbed and all hope for recovery was gone. The lamenters would run through the streets to the *besmedresh*, or house of prayer, pull open the doors to the Holy Ark to expose the Torah scrolls where the Almighty was believed to live, and beg him to save the infirm one from death. When the town's children witnessed this performance, they knew a funeral would take place the next day.[170]

This practice of the "wailing woman" is mentioned in both the Hebrew and Christian bibles. In the ancient Middle East, as well as in some contemporary cultures, the woman who performs the public lament is understood to be helping her community come to terms with their collective grief: "In ancient times, mourning or wailing women were groups of women invited to attend funerals and other sombre events to lead the participants in mourning much like a cantor or choir leads a congregation in its liturgy."[171]

The titles for these women can be translated as "wise women" or "skilled women," names that can be interpreted as meaning that the art of healing through the performance of a mourning ritual was something that had to be learned:

> Wailing women not only had to be able to draw on the reservoir of laments handed down through the generations, but they also had to adapt the laments to suit the particular needs of the current situation. . . . Their laments represent the community's response in the face of extreme trauma.[172]

War and destruction, a normalized part of life in biblical times, affected people directly. By leading their communities in profoundly moving ceremonies, wailing women could swell a community's collective emotions in celebratory victory songs or in sorrowful laments that mourned military defeats. It was in leading public rituals that these wise women brought feelings of unity, empathy, and eventually healing.[173]

This women's healing role was not in any way unique among Ashkenazim of the Pale. Even as late as the twentieth century, the professional woman mourner could be found in many parts of Europe. In southern Italy, for example, the *prefiche* were practicing as late as the 1950s. The Finnish lamenting women of Karelia were considered "honored celebrants," who "developed elaborate rituals for the major rites of passage.... They entered in [to their lament] gradually . . . and gave themselves over to the powers they unleashed and summoned.... In this sense they were more like shamans."[174]

Like Esther-Khaye of Zabludove, these women also conversed with those on the other side of the veil and were "intimate with the energies beyond the common knowledge."[175] And much like the midwife—who, summoned to a birth, immediately sets out to aid those in need—these women were also attentive participants at life's pivotal moments.

Because we are likely never to hear the melodies of the Ashkenazi lamenters such as Esther-Khaye, whose songs were described as causing "even the most cynical of men to cry," this description of a Finnish mourning woman's artistry may provide some insight into the mourning songs of the Pale:

> *Calling upon time honored formulas that are deep inside her she begins to speak in a chanting voice. Her speaking flows with a rhythm. It is rhymed and rich with alliterations. Riding her feelings and drawing from her own deep wellspring of ancient verses and formulations, she pushes off and seeks to find her way into the lament. She addresses both death and the departed. Her voice begins to take on its wailing quality . . . slowly she begins to mix in particular details from the life of the departed.*[176]

These are just a few examples of the Pale's women folk healers, all now gone, having left only faint traces of a path for us to follow. Unlike the ba'alei shem or the male feldshers, women healers such as the opshprekherins never consulted the remedy books. Neither are they believed to have set down their

secret cures in writing. Their ancient traditions, passed orally from one generation to the next, down through the centuries, disappeared along with the healers
themselves. Could it be possible that a literary tradition exists for these women,
and that male scholars have chosen, deliberately or not, to leave these stories
unexplored from their original sources?

Other Medicinal Plant Knowledge

It must be noted that the reliance on herbs was evident in professions beyond
healers in Ashkenazi communities in and outside the Pale prior to the Second
World War. The distillers and tavern keepers present in almost every Eastern
European Ashkenazi town represent another example of medicinal plant knowledge in the Pale. These craftspeople, many of whom emigrated from the Pale
before the Second World War, produced traditional digestive bitters and other
herbal concoctions. For example, the Kantorowicz family established a liqueur
factory in 1823 in Poznan (present-day Poznań, Poland) employing herbs such
as *Gentiana* spp. (gentian) root, *Pimpinella anisum* (anise) seed, and *Acorus
calamus* (calamus) root to infuse their beverages with medicinal qualities.[177]

In addition to the consumption of herbs internally, topical plant preparations
were also common in the Pale. Early twentieth-century American celebrity cos-
metics entrepreneurs, such as Polish émigré Helena Rubinstein, took advantage
of family recipes passed down over generations to create creams and lotions that
promised glowing beauty with proprietary plant-based ingredients.[178] Examples
like these strongly suggest that Ashkenazi knowledge of medicinal herbs was
widespread and deserves more in-depth investigation than the scope of this book.

In Closing: Possibilities

Finally, one question as yet unanswered hangs in the air: why did the Ashkenazim continue to rely on folk practitioners and their old-fashioned plant remedies throughout their years in Eastern Europe until the very end?

In an essay published in 1981, less than four decades after the Second World
War, one Florida researcher innocently pondered something similar: "In our era
of scientific medicine, we may wonder if any folk belief or popular medicine

plant use survives among Jewish people." The answers he received from a few elderly immigrants were, for anyone interested in herbalism among the Ashkenazi ancestors, both astonishing and profoundly heartbreaking—unbeknownst to the researcher, his informants were none other than a handful of the elusive Ashkenazi folk healers who had survived the Second World War:

> An interview sampling of elderly Jews in Miami, Florida, produced some interesting findings . . . they remembered much from their own past, whether in Eastern Europe or recently immigrated to America. A dozen informants described twenty-one different medicinal uses for plants and herbs: . . . garlic placed in the ear for aches, assafetida hung around the neck for contagious diseases, horehound boiled with anise for cough, camomile (sic) flower tea for cramps, malma (mallow) leaf tea for malaise, clover stem suppositories for infants with gas cramps, parsnip as a diuretic, parsley as a deodorant, corn leaf tea for kidney pain, camphor oil for earache, flaxseed poultice for infection and swelling, raw potato slices on burns, dried raspberry for the "grip," castor oil and enemas and cupping "shtetl bankes" for bronchitis.[179]

Even the scant information the researcher gathered from these elders in 1970s Florida reveals how remarkably close their remedies were to what today's herbalists rely on. Many of these same remedies were also mentioned in the informal survey I posted in a social media group devoted to Jewish genealogy—several respondents told of their grandmothers using raw potato slices for healing burns and fevers, garlic for earaches, and many more remembered "bankes," or cupping, for colds and other respiratory ailments. Most remarkably of all, the elderly Ashkenazi immigrants in Florida had reported herbal remedies that matched the findings of the Soviet-era ethnographic survey.

It's difficult to accept that in the decades after the Second World War, folk healers who had survived their ordeals had not been sought out for their traditional knowledge. Not one known ethnobotanical study has ever been undertaken to honor the healers of the Pale. Instead, it's the fragments such as those presented here that must suffice for now. Hopefully these few pages will inspire further research regarding the Pale of Settlement's Ashkenazi folk healers and their herbal remedies.

We hope that a closer survey of the written record that remains will reveal more. In one yizkor book, from the town of Burshtin (present-day Burshtyn, Ukraine), one memoirist recalls the town's Jewish midwife, Fayge di bobe, who delivered most of the town's children in the late nineteenth and early twentieth centuries, until a trained *akusherke* appeared. The author describes some of Fayge's cures: "She had her remedies for all sorts of diseases. A honeycomb for swelling, a hot broth, or a bath of milk and honey for a child with rickets."[180]

Another yizkor book, from the town of Felshtin (present-day Hvardiisk'ke, Ukraine), recounts "mama's unwritten remedy book," including the use of quinine for fever.[181] Similarly a yizkor for Voislavitsa (present-day Wisłowiec, Poland) describes the "*heymishe refu'os*" (domestic remedies) used by women healers, such as foot-soaks in a basin of cold water and ash, and horseradish for headaches.[182]

And the authors of the yizkor book for the shtetl of Antipolye (present-day Antopal', Belarus) note that before the arrival of trained medical professionals around 1850, "All medical care was in the hands of bobes, znachors, 'good Jews' (gute yidn), rabbis, opshprekhers, and 'vaysers.' The 'diagnoses' were simple then: they dealt with 1) illnesses with fever, 2) abdominal pain, 3) wounds, 4) joint and bone fractures, and 5) 'craziness' ("meshugeim")." It's interesting that the authors contrast Slavic *znachors* and Yiddish *vaysers*, the words being cognate, and further distinguish them from the *opshprekhers* (whether male or female)—yet another clue that traditional health care in the Pale was an intercommunal affair, where all community members, regardless of ethnicity or faith, placed their fate in the hands of healers from each group. And why not? The plants don't discriminate but offer support to everyone who seeks and is open to their medicine.[183]

All of which suggests we may still be able recover the ancestral Ashkenazi folk healing traditions embodied by the opshprekherin and the midwife, the mourner and the wet nurse, hiding in plain sight.

In closing, the Florida researcher reminds us how important our connection to the natural world is for remembering our ancestors, for healing ourselves, and for the health of future generations:

> *Botanical medicine has been one small vehicle for carrying the function of culture, to provide continuity with the past through family and community relationships. For Jewish people, often struggling against adverse forces, these common and continuous [herbal] practices helped maintain cohesive identity. Medicinal plants are richly expressive as vehicles for these needs, serving as agents of healing and hope, reflecting our ties to the earth, and showing continuous regrowth with the seasonal cycles.[184]*

PART II
MATERIA MEDICA

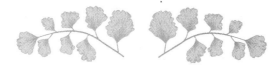

NOTES ON THE *MATERIA MEDICA*

The twenty-six herbs included in this *materia medica* are all plants known by folk healers in towns within the Pale of Settlement with a significant Jewish population between the two world wars (see appendix 1 on page 260).

The Ashkenazi towns and villages where informants were interviewed appear at the end of each relevant plant monograph, and each town is cited by the Yiddish name it was called at the time of the survey. For population statistics between the world wars for each town cited and for present-day town names, see appendix 1.

The Soviet plant surveys, of which the Ukrainian study was a part, appear to closely follow the route taken by the earlier An-Sky ethnographic expeditions through the Pale. It's probable that the Soviet ethnobotanical expeditions drew upon the earlier work by An-Sky fifteen to twenty years earlier as a source for reliable informants, those well versed in the region's folkways and folk medicine.

A further area of interest is the pattern of medicinal plant usage that distinguishes Ashkenazi regions from non-Jewish regions in the Pale. When organized by oblast or province, the Ukrainain survey data show patterns that illustrate which herbs were more relied on by each region, and they can be broken down further by towns with varying degrees of Ashkenazi presence. Though it appears that distinct groups applied specific local plants they found most helpful, more research is needed in this area for a better understanding of what these patterns might mean. We plan to cover this topic in the future.

The *materia medica* for the twenty-six herbs listed here have been traced back as far as Dioscorides and also show their application within the context of herbalism up to the present time. A chronology in appendix 2 (page 263) shows approximate eras of the herbalists, physicians, and botanists cited in each plant profile.

We emphasize plants and their application in Eastern Europe. Plant comparisons are meant to illustrate Eastern European herbal remedies alongside the better-known western European applications—and not only geographically but to draw attention to similarities and differences over time.

Herbs that aren't found documented by Dioscorides but that were present in the towns and villages of the Pale are of particular interest because they leave many questions as yet unanswered. Were they known in Eurasia to peoples other than the Greeks, such as the Tatars, a group many Ashkenazim esteemed above all other folk healers?[1] Or did knowledge of these plants come from the Far East, their healing abilities transmitted via contact among peripatetic groups? Or were the healers in the Pale the first to apply these remedies?

Where use in contemporary countries is mentioned, note there is often a difference between folk medicine and official, state, or government medicine.

The plants listed in this *materia medica* are only a small fraction of those known and employed by Ashkenazim in the Pale up to the Second World War. It should be noted that in addition to the medicinal plants, other healing methods were also popular such as *bankes*, or cupping, and the "guggle-muggle," an egg and milk concoction that was given to children with colds. Another popular remedy was the sock that was placed around the neck of a child with a sore throat at night before bed. And of course chicken soup, the most famous remedy of all, known for centuries and which itself contains medicinal plants, such as dill and root vegetables.

I recall once reading that Ashkenazi medicinal application of plants was mainly in the form of herbal teas. This most certainly is reflected in the many decoctions and infusions reported by the traditional folk healers in the Pale of Settlement.

This *materia medica* is not intended as a usage guide but rather a document of historical interest. If you work with any herbs medicinally, always check reputable sources beforehand and be sure to work with the plants carefully and respectfully.

1

ALOE ARBORESCENS

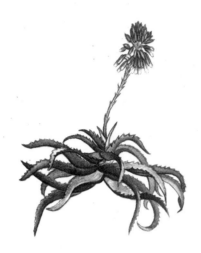

FAMILY: Asphodelaceae

COMMON ENGLISH NAMES: aloe

YIDDISH: אלאע ,אליאיז ,אליאָ

HEBREW: אלואי ,אלווא ,אללוי ,אלווי ,אלוא ,אלוי ,אלי עצי ,אלווי ,אלואי

UKRAINIAN: Алое деревовидне, алоя деревувата, алоя, алоісь, сабур, столітник, столетник, кактус, ранник, каксуль, доктор, рапшіль

GERMAN: Aloe

POLISH: aloes drzewniasty

RUSSIAN: Алое древовидное, столетник, сабур

LITHUANIAN: Medėjantis alavijas

DESCRIPTION AND LOCATION: Perennial, sometimes tree-like plant, native to the semiarid regions of Africa, cultivated in Europe for decorative and medicinal purposes.[1] Narrow leaves are somewhat flat and thick, curl backward, and begin in the upper part of the root. Spine-like teeth on leaf margins protrude slightly. In remote parts of Africa, aloes may grow from thirty to sixty feet in height, the stem sometimes attaining a circumference of ten feet. Red, yellow, or purple tubular flowers grow on erect, terminal spikes and are divided into six narrow segments at the mouth, producing angular seeds and blooms most of the year. Single stalk-like root.[2]

EARLY ALOE REMEDIES: In the Hebrew Bible, "aloes" are described as fragrant, a characteristic that doesn't seem to corroborate what might be said of the plants called "aloe" today. Most likely, biblical aloes were Indian sandalwood (Santalum album) or agarwood, also known as aloeswood, and were derived from a mold-infected Aquilaria tree, which produces a signature aromatic resin to protect itself from the offending pathogen.

The ancient Greeks, on the other hand, identified the aloe plant as having medicinal qualities sufficient to "purge the bowels" or other digestive ailments. They also relied on the plant to mend injuries and cicatrize flesh (heal wounds by way of scar formation); if necessary, the leaf juice was also sought out to reattach a severed foreskin. In Athens aloe was found capable of relieving bleeding hemorrhoids, soothing black eyes, clearing blepharitis (the inflamed tiny oil glands of the inner eyelid), curbing hair loss, soothing tonsil inflammation, and generally supporting oral health.[3]

By the second century CE, Galen had concentrated aloe's medicinal powers to two: loosening the bowels in order to purge rotting matter, and reducing bile and phlegm. He also noted that the juice could act as an effective astringent when applied topically.[4]

In the second millennium, in Germany Hildegard von Bingen recommended a formula of aloe, myrrh, wheat, and poppy, which was to be kneaded into a dough and applied to the head, including the neck and ears, and then covered with a cap as a method for relieving migraine headaches.[5] To cure "worms in the teeth," she described a steam prepared with aloe and myrrh.[6] To strengthen "fevers in the stomach" or relieve a cough, a plaster made with aloe leaf juice was placed upon the navel or chest, respectively. For ague, or fevers accompanied by shivering fits, Hildegard advised mixing horehound juice or powder, depending on the season, with aloe and licorice, which were then cooked in wine and drunk. Jaundice was cured by taking aloe juice diluted with water.[7] She recommended the juice be applied as a topical to ulcers and scabies.[8]

Paracelsus for his part wrote cryptically of aloe combined with myrrh as part of an alchemic recipe for deriving sulfur. With this remarkable preparation, one might expect an "excellent preservative in the plague, in pleurisy, in all abscesses and putridities of the body."[9]

Tobias ha-Kohen (also known as Tobias Cohn) was even more obscure on the subject; he may have used a term for the plant that is unknown today. In his text the single instance of the word that translates as *aloe* appears to deal with ear infections to be treated with an aloe prepared with chamomile.[10]

ALOE ARBORESCENS CONTEMPORARY ACTIONS: emollient, purgative, vulnerary;[11] anti-inflammatory, antiseptic, demulcent, stimulant laxative, soothing[12]

ALOE ARBORESCENS CONTEMPORARY MEDICINAL PARTS: leaves

ALOE IN CONTEMPORARY HERBALISM: World-renowned American herbalist Rosemary Gladstar calls aloe "a virtual first-aid kit in a plant" and recommends readers grow the herb as a houseplant. If one were to require a purgative (a strong laxative), aloe is recommended in powdered or pill form; however, she and other herbalists, both ancient and modern, caution that this should be practiced with care and completely avoided by pregnant or nursing women.[13] The fresh leaves of the plant, opened to expose the juice and applied to a skin irritation, are still known today, as they were to the ancients, as a household remedy. The fresh juice is also known to help wounds by preventing or drawing out infections. To wash wounds or irritated eyes, a tea can also be prepared from fresh aloe leaf juice.[14]

American clinical herbalists Thomas Easley and Steven Horne, and British medical phytotherapists Simon Mills and Kerry Bone, write not only about aloe's fame for soothing skin and mucous membranes but also about the efficacy of its juice for strengthening the immune system to help combat degenerative diseases such as arthritis, cancer, and AIDS, and that the safest preparation is a diluted juice made from the pulp.[15] David Hoffmann, another leading British medical herbalist, notes that in small doses the plant can bring on menstruation; he cautions that aloe should be avoided during pregnancy and nursing, as it's excreted in mother's milk and could serve as a purgative to a nursing infant.[16]

In Germany the fresh leaf of the aloe plant is recommended as a laxative, while the dried, powdered herb is a component of the well-loved Swedish bitters elixir recipe.[17]

Russians have also grown aloe in their homes for many years; for skin irritations they apply the fresh leaf topically on an affected area. Internally the fresh juice is used as a remedy for digestive issues. In the early twentieth century, the Russian surgeon and ophthalmologist Vladimir Filatov found that the leaves, when stored in the dark at low temperatures, underwent a biological transformation that produced substances that stimulate the body's "vital processes." Commercial preparations derived by this method have proven internally effective at stimulating the immune system and addressing respiratory ailments. Russian dermatologists, ophthalmologists, and gynecologists currently use aloe-derived topical preparations; as elsewhere, Russian medical professionals caution against aloe use during pregnancy.[18]

Cultivated aloes in Poland are brought indoors to survive the harsh Eastern European winters.[19] The plant is also one of twenty-seven herbs that make up a traditional recipe for a homemade benedictine (herbal liqueur). The entire formula is generally a closely guarded secret, but some of the other known herbal ingredients include angelica root, calamus root, cinnamon, orange peel, ginger, oranges, vanilla, nutmeg, saffron, and cloves.[20]

Aloe is a very common houseplant in Lithuania as well. It's also a remedy used in the official government-sanctioned medicine of that country. During the Second World War, the juice from the leaves was used to treat wounds and sores that took longer to heal. Lithuanian medicine uses the plant's juice to treat chronic gastritis, improve appetite, and strengthen the immune system. A syrup made from the plant is taken to cure anemia. Aloe is also used for skin conditions including healing after radiation therapy, dermatitis, eczema, psoriasis, and neurodermatitis. Folk medicine practitioners mix the fresh leaf juice with lard, butter, and cocoa to treat pulmonary infections and chronic bronchitis.[21]

In Ayurvedic medicine, the traditional medicine of India, many species of aloe are regarded as healing. The plant is known to have cooling properties, while its flavor properties are considered bitter, astringent, pungent, and sweet. The aloe's medicine in Ayurveda is extremely varied. Among its many strengths, aloe is known to support the liver, spleen, blood, digestion, and skin health. It's also sought to relieve anemia, asthma, and constipation. In addition aloe is known as *kumari*, "virgin," and is a main tonic for restoring women's reproductive health.[22]

ALOE IN EARLY TWENTIETH-CENTURY EUROPEAN HERBALISM: Early twentieth-century European ethnographers confirmed that the juice of various plants belonging to the aloe genus was still being used as a laxative, continuing the ancient tradition. They also learned of its application as a gastric strengthening agent in Indian folk medicine. Additionally its use as an abortifacient was documented—when taken internally it can cause uterine contractions.[23]

The classic *A Modern Herbal* reiterates aloe's strength as a "purgative for those of sedentary habits and phlegmatic constitutions," adding that because its action is mainly on the large intestine, it is also helpful as a vermifuge, with the caveat that caution should be observed as the herb could induce hemorrhoids.[24]

In Russian folk medicine, the fresh juice of the aloe leaves was used externally for wound healing, boils, and herpes infections, and internally for tuberculosis and headache.[25]

***ALOE ARBORESCENS* IN ASHKENAZI HERBALISM IN THE PALE IN THE EARLY TWENTIETH CENTURY:** In Apt, Poland, before the Second World War, at least one matriarch kept an aloe plant on the window sill. With fresh juice from its leaves, she would treat minor cuts, burns, and boils by applying it directly on an affected area. This remedy was also known to open the wound and draw the pus, thereby preventing infection. Children in the Pale were taught this healing technique and a few others that today have become more obscure. One of these—fresh, clean cobwebs, especially those found in barns—was a healing device that had been used for centuries and continued to be reliable to both clean and bandage minor cuts. The webs were wrapped on the wound to staunch the bleeding. If cobwebs weren't available, a quick pee on the affected area was also known to disinfect in a pinch.[26]

In Ashkenazi communities of the Pale at the turn of the twentieth century, the fresh plant juice and the leaves, cleaned of thorns and cut into small pieces, were boiled with honey. This mixture was a widely used remedy for tuberculosis of the lungs, particularly in Polona and Letichev.

Folk healers in Letichev also looked to this same preparation for treating colds and catarrhs of the stomach and as a remedy for tuberculosis of the throat.[27]

2

ARISTOLOCHIA CLEMATITIS

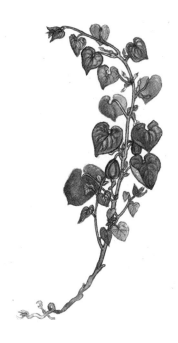

FAMILY: Aristolochiaceae

COMMON ENGLISH NAMES: Aristolochia root, birthwort

YIDDISH: צ׳יבעך*

HEBREW: ארטכלס, אריסטולוחיא״ה לוננ״ה, אריסטולוחיא״ה רוטונד״ה אזניות

---

* Schaechter cites this name for "Dutchman's pipe," not necessarily *A. clematitis*. However, we suspect that the names філійник, філильник ("filijnyk," "filyl'nyk") attested in towns with large Jewish populations, viz., Monasterishtche and Zhitomir, may reflect a pronunciation of Ukrainian хвилівник by non-Ukrainian (i.e., Yiddish) speakers.

UKRAINIAN: Хвилівник звичайний, хвилівник, хвилильник, філійник, хвилійник, філильник, хвилінник, хвилейник, котові яйця

GERMAN: Gewöhnliche Osterluzei, aufrechte Osterluzei

POLISH: Kokornak powojnikowy, kokornak powojnikowaty

RUSSIAN: Кирказон обыкновенный, кирказон ломоносовидный

LITHUANIAN: Kartuolė

DESCRIPTION AND LOCATION: Perennial herb that grows along fences, undergrowth, edges of fields, and vineyards. Its sinuous stem can reach a height of three feet and is upright and yellow-green with dark green, bean-shaped leaves. Clusters of light green tubular flowers bloom May–June. A long, thin, fleshy yet brittle root appears grayish on the outside, brownish-yellow on the inside. The plant has a bitter taste and a strong disagreeable odor when fresh.[28]

***ARISTOLOCHIA CLEMATITIS* EARLY REMEDIES:** Early medicinal documentation of Aristolochia goes back to the ancient Egyptians, who found the plant helpful in treating snakebites.[29]

As a medicinal plant, birthwort has been much written about over the centuries. Most controversial has been its use in women's health, for it is highly toxic, and can be potentially dangerous. Depending on the prevailing philosophical or religious thought at the time of their writing, men who documented this plant's role in gynecological health either wrote extensively about it or left it out completely. It was women folk healers, such as midwives, who over the centuries quietly passed along their understanding of the herb's relationship with the female body from one generation to the next.[30]

Dioscorides identifies two distinct types, the round and the long. The variety described as round was a remedy for deadly poisons, including snakebites, and was helpful for asthma relief, hiccups, shivering, spleen support, relaxing spasms, and soothing pains in the side; when applied as a poultice, birthwort could remove stuck thorns and needles from the flesh. It also cleaned the teeth and gums. The variety described as long was known to draw out matter compacted from the uterus of a woman in labor, or when applied in a pessary could remove an embryo or fetus.[31]

Hildegard confusingly described *"byverwurtz"* as both hot and also somewhat cold. She recommended pulverizing the dried root and leaves then mixing them with powders of feverfew and cinnamon to keep "great or lasting illness" away for the rest of one's life. To conserve the medicine for later use, she advised storing it in a closed earthen vessel that was to be buried in the ground.[32]

Maimonides was of the opinion that the round variety, which in his time was imported from Mesopotamia (present-day Iraq), was more effective than the long. He gave the plant's name in Persian as *"zarawand"* and in Spanish as *"calabazuela,"* and he emphasized that the original Greek name was given to signify the emmenagogic action of the root.[33]

German herbals of the fifteenth century recommend *Aristolochia clematitis* for the relief of gout, and in powder form for the treatment of wounds; combined with aloe in the form of a plaster, it was deployed against cancer, fistulas, lupus, and leprosy. Later, in the sixteenth century, German botanist Adam Lonicer recommended applying the plant in cases of external fractures and wounds.[34]

By the seventeenth century the plant's dried root was a constituent in the famous Duke of Portland Powder. Along with equal parts of the leaves of *Ajuga chamaepitys* (yellow bugle), the leaves and tops of *Erythraea centaurium* (common centaury) and *Teucrium chamaedrys* (wall germander), and the roots of *Gentiana lutea* (great yellow gentian), the mixture was believed to be a remedy for gout.[35]

In the eighteenth century, as a remedy listed in the chapter "Malignant Fevers," the Swiss physician Samuel-Auguste Tissot included in his medical text a *"Teriaca pauperum,"* or poor man's treacle, to bring about a speedy recovery.[36] His formula No. 42 consisted of equal parts root of birthwort, elecampane, and myrrh, plus conserve of juniper berries, all compounded into an electuary finished off with a syrup of orange peel.[37]

The physician Tobias ha-Kohen also wrote of the two Aristolochias, and in his section on women's health he harkens back to the ancient Greeks by identifying both the round and the long plants as helpful in childbirth.[38]

ARISTOLOCHIA CLEMATITIS **CONTEMPORARY ACTIONS:** diaphoretic, emmenagogue, febrifuge, oxytocic, stimulant

ARISTOLOCHIA CLEMATITIS **CONTEMPORARY MEDICINAL PARTS:** entire plant

ARISTOLOCHIA CLEMATITIS **IN CONTEMPORARY HERBALISM:** Because of its toxic and extremely dangerous properties, this plant has fallen out of favor in contemporary herbalism. In the latter half of the twentieth century, one American herbalist wrote of the plant's efficacy internally for stomach complaints and menstrual irregularities and externally as a decoction used as a wash to treat wounds and leg ulcers. However, it was also cautioned that any use of the plant be done under strict medical supervision.[39]

ARISTOLOCHIA CLEMATITIS **IN EUROPEAN HERBALISM IN THE EARLY TWENTIETH CENTURY:** In her classic reference, *A Modern Herbal*, Maude Grieve wrote of *A. clematitis, A. rotunda,* and *A. longa* as all still being retained in the official herbal catalogues of Europe, where the plants are indigenous. She singles out *A. clematitis,* or birthwort, as "found in England, usually near old ruins, as if it had been cultivated for its medical use, as an aid to parturition," that is, in childbirth.[40]

In Russia birthwort was widely used in folk medicine, in particular for vomiting, cough, pulmonary tuberculosis, scurvy, and gout, and as a diuretic.[41]

The most interesting finding on birthwort comes to us from a European nineteenth-century ethnobotanical study that noted: "Hemorrhoids are little known among the Ruthenes; the most reported cases come from the nobles and the Jews." This study then elaborates several remedies for the condition. One of these indicates a tea for non-bleeding hemorrhoids that was to be brewed from Aristolochia.[42]

ARISTOLOCHIA CLEMATITIS **IN ASHKENAZI HERBALISM IN THE PALE IN THE EARLY TWENTIETH CENTURY:** Aristolochia was a common plant in the Pale of the early twentieth century and could be found in woods, especially those that flooded in spring, as well as amidst shrubs, along ravines, and in orchards; it was largely absent on the left bank of the Dnieper River, where Ashkenazi settlements were not as common as on the right bank. Interestingly the plant was not reported to have been used in gynecological health in these communities. Rather, earlier German remedies for healing wounds with this plant are echoed in the folk medicine of the Pale.

In Uman, located on the right bank of the river and well situated within the Pale of Settlement, a leaf infusion of the plant was given by folk healers there for non-bleeding hemorrhoids.

Patients suffering from rheumatism were bathed in a decoction of the whole plant in Romen and Uman.

A combination of birthwort's fresh leaves, or its dried, ground leaves or steamed leaves (occasionally mixed with sour cream), rootstocks, and leaf juice constituted a treatment for wounds, mainly festering sores, abscesses, and boils. This remedy was popular among the folk healers of the Pale most notably in the towns of Kiev, Romen, Uman, Monasterishtche, Cherkoss, and Bohslov.

A decoction of *Aristolochia clematitis*, *Bryonia alba* (white bryony), and *Lathyrus niger* (black pea) was used internally and externally for the treatment of nervous disorders by a folk healer in Birzula.

In Yelisavetgrod fresh leaf juice or a fresh leaf decoction was used as a wash to rid the head of lice.

In folk veterinary medicine a powder made of the leaves or of the dried whole plant was sprinkled on wounds infected by worms in the settlements of both Yelisavetgrod and Bohslov.

A leaf decoction was also used to wash animals with excessive itching in Broslev.[43]

3

ARTEMISIA ABSINTHIUM

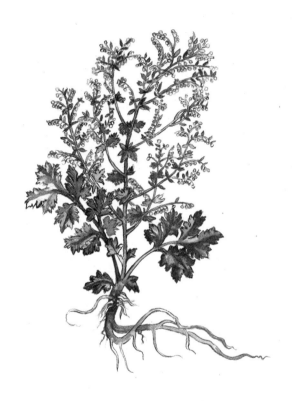

FAMILY: Asteraceae

COMMON ENGLISH NAMES: wormwood, grand wormwood, absinthe, absinthium, absinthe wormwood

YIDDISH: ביטערגראָז, ביטערער פּאָלין, ווערעמקרויט, פּאָלון, פּאָלוו

HEBREW: האבסינט, לענה

UKRAINIAN: Полин звичайний, полин гіркий, полинь, полинь пахнюча, полин, полинець, адже пелин

GERMAN: Wermut

POLISH: Bylica piołun

RUSSIAN: Полынь горькая

LITHUANIAN: Pelynas, kartusis kietis, pelūnas, metėlis, kartėlis

DESCRIPTION AND LOCATION: From the perennial root of *Artemisia absinthium* grow firm, branching stems, which are woody at their base. When in bloom, the plant's whitish stem, which can reach two and a half feet, becomes covered with fine silky hairs. Leaves, also covered with this fuzz, grow up to three inches long and one and one half inches across; they are indented in repeated segments, each segment being both narrow and blunt. Small, globe-shaped greenish-yellow flowers bloom from July to October. Both the leaves and flowers have a bitter taste and characteristic scent that have been described as "very green," sharp, bitter, and herbaceous.[44] The root also has a "warm" and aromatic flavor. *Artemisia absinthium* is native to the temperate regions of Eurasia and North Africa and is widely naturalized in the northern part of North America.[45]

ARTEMISIA ABSINTHIUM EARLY REMEDIES: As a medicinal plant, wormwood has a very long and illustrious history, which doubtless predates its recorded use. The herb is likely mentioned in the Egyptian Ebers Papyrus (1600 BCE) as the oldest medicinal and cultivated plant. While the flora described in the papyrus seems very similar to *Artemisia absinthium,* it cannot be determined whether this is so. In ninth-century Europe the first verifiable reference to *Artemesia absinthium* was recorded in Walafridus Strabus's *Hortulus,* then several hundred years later by the German abbess and herbalist Hildegard von Bingen.[46]

Meanwhile, religious scholars have written that the Hebrew Bible refers to the plant, identifying it by its intensely bitter taste, which most likely accounts for wormwood's association with gall as a symbol of bitter calamity and sorrow. One twentieth-century work on biblical botany offered this summation of the symbolic religious association for Bronze Age Jews: "Oriental people usually typify sorrow, cruelty, and calamity of any kind by plants of a poisonous nature. Since the Hebrews considered all bitter-tasting plants to be poisonous, the 'root of wormwood' and the 'wormwood and the gall' would offer to them a most emphatic and unmistakable metaphor."[47]

The genus *Artemisia* is named for Artemis, the Greek goddess of the hunt, the moon, and chastity, and, over time, has also become associated with childbirth and nature.

Dioscorides wrote that wormwood's character is warm and astringent. Its numerous powers include its ability to clear "bilious elements" that pass through the intestinal tract, its ability to counteract nausea, and its actions as a diuretic, a carminative, and an appetite stimulant. He recommended it be used to treat jaundice, and in gynecological conditions wormwood was known to "draw down the menses both when drunk and when used topically with honey."[48]

Wormwood in vinegar was an antidote for poisonings from toadstools, hemlock, the bite of the shrew mouse, and the bite of the great weever, also known as the "sea dragon." In addition the herb, when taken with honey, would heal sore throats, pustules that were more painful at night, black eyes and dim-sightedness, not to mention purulent ears. As a decoction, inhaling the steam was helpful for earaches, and reduced down with grape syrup, it was applied as a poultice for very painful eyes. Mixed with rose ointment, it was plastered on the stomach for digestive complaints. This same preparation was also suitable for treating edema and spleen conditions. In the summer it was drunk as an aperitif to bring good health.

In addition to these medical applications, the ancient Greeks protected their fabrics from insect infestation by sprinkling wormwood in their storage cabinets, from whence came the common English name for the plant. An oil infusion was made from wormwood to be rubbed into the skin as a mosquito repellent. Wormwood-infused oil was sprinkled on books to protect them from mice as well.[49]

In the tenth century Avicenna extolled the herb's virtues for healing eye inflammations, gall bladder complaints, and menstrual disorders among other treatments.[50]

By the twelfth century in Germany, the abbess and herbalist Hildegard von Bingen had recorded a wormwood recipe that included vervain to dispel any toothache that was brought about by putrid blood or discharges originating in the brain. This decoction was to be both applied as a poultice on the jaw where the affected tooth was embedded and simultaneously taken internally with wine.[51]

For "incontinence" Hildegard recommended that a man "so excited with pleasure that the foam reaches his organ of ejaculation but is for some reason stopped and retained inside the body," should he become sick from his inability, drink a warm mixture of wormwood and rue juice, combined with sugar, honey, and wine, but only after having a bite to eat.[52]

Hildegard described "*wermuda*," the vernacular German word for wormwood at the time, as very warm and strong and as the main remedy for all sorts of ailments. For headache an infusion of the plant in warm wine was applied as a poultice around the head and neck overnight. In an infused oil it was rubbed on the chest to help with a cough, or any pain, to heal both internally and externally. For gout she recommended that a mixture of wormwood with deer tallow and bone marrow be anointed on the patient. This same combination could be warmed with honey and wine and drunk intermittently from late spring to early autumn to assist with "melancholy, clear eyes, [to] strengthen heart and lungs, warm the stomach, and clear the intestines for better digestion."[53]

In medieval Poland the remedy books advised herbalists to make their treatments more effective by refreshing their wormwood remedies. This could be accomplished by replacing old leaves once their strong odor had worn off. In the sixteenth century the Polish botanist Simon Syreniusz wrote that wormwood "warms a cold stomach and awakens the appetite," reiterating the ancient Greek literature. An infusion of the herb was recommended to treat any stomach disorders; and a decoction of the leaves as a compress relieved burning eyes. A more unique remedy for injuries called for egg white to be combined with fresh chopped wormwood leaves and applied to the bruised area. And in another twist on the plant's ancient legacy, medieval Poles added a solution made from the plant directly into their ink, thus preventing hungry mice and insects from destroying their books. In some parts of Poland fresh leaves were placed beneath the sheets and sprinkled around the bed to discourage fleas. And for livestock *Artemisia* bouquets were hung on the barn door to keep out flies.[54]

In Russia wormwood was used to heal wounds and cleanse the blood—especially when picked in May.[55]

Published in 1577, this verse offers a litany of the accolades wormwood continued to enjoy with healers of the era:

While Wormwood hath seed get a handful or twaine

To save against March, to make flea to refraine:

Where chamber is sweeped and Wormwood is strowne,

What saver is better (if physick be true)

For places infected than Wormwood and Rue?

It is a comfort for hart and the braine

And therefore to have it it is not in vaine.[56]

By the mid to late eighteenth century, Tissot had published his best-selling *Advice to the People,* which included two recipes featuring wormwood in treatments for fevers. The first, No. 37, combined the herb with "Ground Oak" (Chamaedrys or germander), the lesser centaury (*Centaurium pulchellum*), and chamomile (*Matricaria chamomilla*) in tincture form,[57] and it was taken for "putrid" or recurring fevers as a substitute remedy when the preferred formula was not available.[58]

The second of his formulations that included wormwood was No. 43,[59] which was a trio of equal parts lesser centaury, wormwood, and myrrh (*Commiphora*), all powdered, plus a conserve of juniper berries (*Juniperus*) and an additional syrup of wormwood that was to be stirred to a thick consistency and taken for "Intermittent Fevers."[60]

By the time the physician Tobias ha-Kohen set down his recommendations in Hebrew, wormwood's virtues were already well documented throughout western Europe. His views reiterated the plant's ability to stimulate an appetite after fever, its facility for removing internal parasites, and its helpfulness in lowering temperatures. He also recommended formulations with honey, and included *Hypericum* (St. John's wort) and barley in one of the treatments for digestive issues.[61]

ARTEMISIA ABSINTHIUM **CONTEMPORARY ACTIONS:** tonic, stomachic, febrifuge, anthelmintic

ARTEMISIA ABSINTHIUM CONTEMPORARY MEDICINAL PARTS: whole plant

ARTEMISIA ABSINTHIUM IN CONTEMPORARY HERBALISM: The romantic mystique of absinthe, a liqueur made from *Artemisia absinthium*, still lingers in the popular imagination. For almost a century, production and consumption of the elixir was banned, first in the United States and then in France, because it was associated with deviant behavior and ill health.

Today this herb, like so many formerly revered medicinal plants, can be found growing wild in temperate regions throughout the world, utterly unrecognized and ignored by the casual passersby. To the modern herbalist, however, as a medicinal plant wormwood is appreciated for its strong antiparasitic application as well as its digestive and appetite-stimulating abilities. But traditional healers also respect its powerful effects and caution that it should not be taken by pregnant women, nursing mothers, or those with weakened health. Even under the best conditions, the plant should only be used for short periods and preferably as a small part of a larger formulation.[62]

To this day in some rural areas of Wales and across scattered counties in England, *Artemisia absinthium* continues to be one of the most widely used of all contemporary herbal medicines, especially for digestive concerns. It is also still used in some regions as an insecticide, and in others it's deployed against intestinal worms. Less commonly, some have valued the herb as a disinfectant, a tonic and purifier of the body, a rheumatic treatment, a kidney trouble remedy, to relieve colic (in conjunction with elderberry syrup), to help with sleep, and to address diabetes. In Ireland, wormwood as a folk medicine is less in evidence—with the exception of three recorded contemporary cases: a remedy for stomach pain, an insecticide, and a treatment for epilepsy.[63]

In Poland, as in most of the continent, the herb can still be found growing in wastelands and along roadsides as well as established gardens. Poles bathe their pets in a concentrated solution of wormwood to eliminate fleas and have observed that bees avoid areas where the herb grows.[64]

In contemporary Lithuania commercially prepared medicines made with *Artemisia absinthium* are available for appetite stimulants, gastric and duodenal ulcers, glandular health, bronchial asthma, eczema, rheumatism, and to stimulate nonspecific immunity. The plant's essential oil has been found to have properties close to camphor and is thought to improve cardiovascular and nervous system health.

In Lithuanian folk medicine, for yeast infections a poultice dressing has been advised with equal parts wormwood and medicinal sage. And for intestinal worms the blossoms are taken in a tea every two hours for two to three days. To stimulate the appetite or to increase bile secretion, a mixture of wormwood and poppy is recommended. For appetite stimulation, improvement of digestion, and treatment of chronic gastritis, wormwood is added, as part of a larger herbal formula, to one glass of boiling water and taken in amounts of one to two tablespoons two to three times a day before meals. Regular consumption of the plant is warned against, as it could lead to poisoning. The Lithuanian spirits industry includes wormwood in its liqueur and vodka products.[65]

ARTEMISIA ABSINTHIUM IN EUROPEAN HERBALISM IN THE EARLY TWENTIETH CENTURY: With the exception of rue, wormwood is the bitterest European herb known; prior to hops, it was by far the most used by brewers to flavor their beer.

In Britain in the early twentieth century, wormwood was seen as a nervine tonic and particularly helpful for "the falling sickness," as epilepsy was then known. It was also regarded as a good remedy for weak digestion, debility, and flatulence.

Different parts of the plant were applied to different ailments. The juice of the larger leaves that grow from the root at the base of the stalk was a remedy for jaundice and edema, although this remedy caused nausea. A fresh, light infusion of the tops of the plant eased disorders of the stomach, stimulated the appetite, strengthened digestion, and prevented sickness after meals.

For a vermifuge the flowers, dried and powdered, were very effective against these pests, and they were also the best choice to treat a fever with shivering.

The plant's intensely bitter, tonic, and stimulant qualities at that time recommended wormwood not only as an ingredient in medicinal preparations but also for various liqueurs, of which the notorious "absinthe" was the most popular. Vermouth takes its name from the herb and has been known as a preserver of the mind—from its medicinal characteristics as a nervine and mental restorative. If not ingested habitually, it has been understood to soothe spinal pain and calm those with anxiety issues.

By the time Maude Grieve published her herbal in the 1930s, the drug absinthium—which was included in the *British Pharmacopoeia* as an extract, infusion, and tincture—was rarely used; Grieve speculated it might be of value in nervous diseases such as neurasthenia, because it was thought to stimulate the cerebral hemispheres, specifically the cortex cerebri. She cautioned, however, when taken in excess it produced lightheadedness and epileptic convulsions.[66]

Warnings against the use of this plant are included in all of the literature of the early twentieth century. For example, a German source counseled, "In large quantities it is very dangerous because cramps develop; chronic usage also leads to various types of damage to the central nervous system, such as convulsions, stupefaction, etc. If ingested occasionally, it does no harm."[67] Ukrainian sources were less circumspect: wormwood should not be abused, particularly with anemia. Prolonged or excessive use of wormwood, even in low doses, may lead to seizures, convulsions, hallucinations, or insanity.[68]

In other parts of western Europe in the early twentieth century, absinthe played a major role in the production of schnapps, particularly in France. In Italy wormwood wine was considered an excellent appetite stimulant and was often drunk in the morning, especially by convalescents. In Dalmatia a decoction of absinthe (*pelinj*) was considered to be a safe remedy for menopausal fever; it was also still widely used as a gastric remedy in scientific and folk medicine in parts of Europe during this period.[69]

In early twentieth-century Russian folk medicine, a decoction was used for intermittent fevers, meteorism, liver colic, appendicitis, and intestinal catarrhs and as an anthelmintic. Compresses were used externally for bruises and abscesses. Another source adds that the herb was also taken orally in powders and vodka extracts to stimulate the appetite, digestion, and as a carminative.[70]

ARTEMISIA ABSINTHIUM IN ASHKENAZI HERBALISM IN THE PALE IN THE EARLY TWENTIETH CENTURY:[71] In the Pale *Artemisia absinthium* was ubiquitous, growing in villages, forests, and fields, and traditional healers of the region were familiar with this plant and its numerous virtues.

In the dozen settlements of Anapol, Polona, Ritzev, Lachovitz, Olt-Kosntin, Monasterishtche, Broslev, Zvenigorodka, Zaslov, Chopovitch, Balte, and Bohslov, a decoction or tincture of the entire herb or of its leaves and flowers was taken as a remedy for stomach ailments such as diarrhea, bloody diarrhea, or dysentery. And following in the footsteps of the ancients and also of Russian traditional usage, these folk healers offered the formula to stimulate appetite and digestion as well.

In Broslev, Litin, and Balte a tincture of the whole plant or its young leaves was used by healers in the treatment of cholera, an infectious disease brought on by ingesting contaminated food or water, which causes severe watery diarrhea and can lead to dehydration and even death if untreated.

In Lachovitz a whole-plant infusion was taken or applied topically to an infected area to treat inflamed gums.

A similar decoction was given as the age-old vermifuge remedy in Kresilev, Anapol, Olt-Kosntin, Zaslav, and Ritzev.

In Monasterishtche, Korosten, and Broslev a whole-plant decoction or a lighter infusion was drunk for head colds, cough, and pain in the chest. It is worth noting that these are exactly the symptoms Hildegard von Bingen, over seven hundred years earlier, had identified as being relieved by treatment with wormwood.

In many towns and villages of the Pale wormwood formulations were a specific folk remedy to combat malaria, both as an intermittent fever and also when the disease manifested as headache. This may have been what Tissot was referring to when he suggested his formulas No. 37 and 43 for the treatment of "intermittent" or "putrid" fevers. In the Pale, to address these symptoms a decoction or tincture of the herb, young leaves, flowers, or (rarely) roots were included. The typical proportion was one plant (fresh or dried) to a half to five glasses of water, of which a half to one glass was taken twice a day on an empty stomach, or two to three hours before a flare-up was anticipated. The large number of settlements found to use this formulation included Slovita, Barditchev, Bohslov, Cherkoss, Korsn, Monasterishtche, and Broslev.

An herb decoction was also employed as a remedy for epilepsy in Monasterishtche. This application of the herb is comparable to what British herbalists had recognized as wormwood's ability to help those suffering from "the falling sickness."

Of all the settlements surveyed between the world wars, only Cherkoss reported that a leaf and flower tincture was drunk by women to induce abortion, recalling the ancient Greeks' knowledge of wormwood's powers.[72]

While this application of an herbal remedy may seem difficult to imagine, many women chose to terminate pregnancies for a variety of reasons. In Poland, for example, prostitution was not illegal, and one memoir that recounts the prostitutes in the small town of Apt suggests a vocational rationale for such extreme measures.[73] Another memoir from Lithuania recalls the need for birth control in the early twentieth century; it's very probable some methods were not always effective, creating a necessity for other means including the choice to end a pregnancy. In Eishyshok, for example, the pharmacist "was known as a tight-lipped man who could be trusted with secrets. He was the one they went to for birth control and other intimate products."[74]

In Monasterishtche and Broslev infants were bathed in a decoction of the herb to relieve their stomachaches.

In official Russian medicine at the time, according to local physicians in Birzula and Balte, in a number of malaria cases a combined treatment of *Artemisia absinthium* with quinine had proven to be very successful when quinine alone had failed to help. In Balte malaria was treated with a wormwood herb decoction for three days; on the fourth day the patient was given a decoction of *Eupatorium cannabinum* (hemp agrimony); in Chopovitch *Sambucus ebulus* (danewort or dwarf elderberry) was occasionally added to this brew.[75]

4

CHELIDONIUM MAJUS

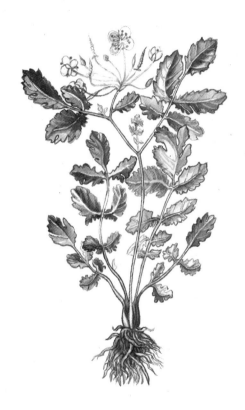

FAMILY: Papaveraceae

COMMON ENGLISH NAMES: greater celandine, nipplewort, swallowwort, tetterwort

YIDDISH: געלזאָפֿט, שׂוואַדענגמילקה, צוכטל, גראַיזער שוואַלבן-מילעך

HEBREW: זילידוניא

UKRAINIAN: Чистотіл, чистотіл більший, бородавник, молочне зілля, жовтець, живе зілля, жовто-зілля, жовте зілля, ранник, йод, росторопша, целідонія, целідоній

GERMAN: Schöllkraut, Goldwurz

POLISH: Glistnik jaskółcze ziele

RUSSIAN: Чистотел большой, бородавник

LITHUANIAN: Didžioji ugniažolė

DESCRIPTION AND LOCATION: Perennial with a thick, fleshy root and a slender, rounded, slightly hairy stem that can attain a height of three feet. Greater celandine is native to Europe and western Asia and has been widely introduced in North America. The branches attach to the stem at slightly swollen junctures, from which they can easily be broken off. Its graceful, somewhat hairy, thinly textured leaves are a pale yellowish-green on top and almost gray beneath, and range from six to twelve inches long and two to three inches wide. Each leaf is divided down the main rib, creating the appearance of two pairs of leaflets opposite each other, with a leaflet at the end. Leaflets have rounded toothlike edges. Flowers bloom through the summer and are arranged at the end of the stem on loose, umbrella-shaped clusters, which eventually turn into long and narrow pods that hold blackish seeds. The whole plant emits a bright orange latex, especially when bruised or broken, has a strong unpleasant odor and nauseating taste, and is a powerful irritant.[76]

CHELIDONIUM MAJUS **EARLY REMEDIES:** In the first century Dioscorides noted that chelidonium was named after the swallow, because the plant grows when their flocks appear and dies back when they depart. He also wrote that adult female swallows fed their blind fledglings with this herb to restore their impaired eyesight.[77]

Galen, not long after, confirmed these early observations, adding that the plant discharges a juice the color of saffron that was drunk for both "yellow and black jaundice," and that "mixed with eye-salves, it clears up dim-sightedness."[78]

Maimonides identified one type of chelidonium in Arabic as *baqlat al-hatatif*, which translates into English as the "plant of swallows." Another he called *al-urug as-sufr*, "yellow roots." Their virtues lay in their ability to sharpen the vision, treat jaundice, soothe shingles, and stop toothaches.[79]

By the late twelfth century, Hildegard von Bingen's observations regarding chelidonium had diverged from the plant's ancient applications. She described *"grintwurtz,"* as it was known during her era, as very warm with a poisonous juice that was both dark and bitter. She understood chelidonium as being too bitter to be successful as a remedy because even if it healed in one area, it would bring greater internal sickness elsewhere in the body. She underscored this by cautioning against ingesting the plant, which she thought would cause ulcers, making digestion painful and unhealthy. Should someone become outwardly infected, however, she recommended the following external cure:

> *Let whoever eats, drinks or touches anything unclean so that they get ulcers on their body, take old fat, add some celandine juice to it, pound these and this dissolve in a dish and rub themselves with this ointment.*[80]

By the late Middle Ages, celandine, the corrupted English pronunciation of the original Greek, was being used medicinally throughout Europe. In the fourteenth century a drink made from the herb was taken for blood health. In the Netherlands the Dutch botanist Carolus Clusius wrote that the juice from greater celandine would rapidly cure "small green wounds," and as an eye medication the herb could remove specks and halt "incipient suffusions."[81]

In the first half of the sixteenth century, the iconoclastic Swiss physician and alchemist Paracelsus, who tested many medical theories that had persisted since the ancient Greeks, wrote that alchemists believed chelidonium could cure jaundice because of its bright yellow color.[82] Early modern scientists had experimented with the herb by pressing out its juice, reducing the liquid down by boiling, and then placing the brew in the sun in the hope that it might transmute into mercury. But these experiments, Paracelsus explains, were done in vain.[83] Despite its disappointing alchemical outcomes, however, Paracelsus included celandine as one of the herbs in a recipe for an "Oil of Arcanum," along with honey, juniper, and oil of flax with sulfur.[84]

Later in the century the well-regarded English botanist John Gerard, possibly unaware of Paracelsus's work, reiterated the findings of the Greeks:

> *The juice of the herbe is good to sharpen the sight, for it cleanseth and cons-*
> *umeth away slimie things that cleave about the ball of the eye and hinder the*

sight and especially being boiled with honey in a brasen vessell, as Dioscorides teacheth.[85]

In the British Isles celandine was also used for bilious and migraine headaches and hemorrhoids, in addition to treating liver conditions.[86]

By the eighteenth century, Swiss physician Samuel-Auguste Tissot echoed Hildegard's earlier writings on celandine's affinity as an external remedy. In possibly its first mention in this role, Tissot recommended the herb as part of a formula to rid oneself of warts: "By drying, or, as it were, withering them up by some moderately corroding Application, such as that of the milky Juice of Purslain, of Fig-leaves, of Chelidonium (Swallow-wort) or of Spurge."[87]

The physician Tobias ha-Kohen, possibly influenced by the writings of Hildegard, included celandine or "zilidonia" in his preferred treatments for topical skin disorders.[88]

CHELIDONIUM MAJUS **CONTEMPORARY ACTIONS:** hepatic, choleretic, cholagogue, antispasmodic, aperient, anti-inflammatory, antiviral, topical vulnerary

CHELIDONIUM MAJUS **CONTEMPORARY MEDICINAL PARTS:** rootstock, herb

CHELIDONIUM MAJUS **IN CONTEMPORARY HERBALISM:** In contemporary Britain medical herbalists use preparations of the aerial, or above-ground, parts of *Chelidonium majus* to assist with liver and gall function, help relieve spasms of the smooth muscles of the gastrointestinal tract, and stimulate the flow of bile. Due to its antimicrobial and antifungal properties, latex from the herb has been used topically for wart removal and to reduce benign tumors, both externally and possibly internally as well. In contemporary British clinical trials, irritable bowel syndrome and colonic polyposis have been among those conditions found to be supported by use of the plant. In traditional Chinese medicine (TCM), the plant is also formulated for similar purposes in addition to support for respiratory ailments such as bronchitis and whooping cough.[89] Some American herbalists, however, strongly caution that "the juice can produce poisoning by congesting the lungs and liver and by narcotic action on the nervous system. Skin poisoning has also resulted from handling the crushed plant."[90]

In recent years Russian medicine has looked to this plant for its actions as an anodyne, anti-inflammatory, antispasmodic, cholagogue, diaphoretic, diuretic, hydragogue, emetic, and topical vulnerary. Official state medicine includes an ointment prepared from the stem's orange latex for the removal of warts, freckles, corns, and fungal infections. One contemporary researcher found that the herb inhibits the growth of cancerous skin cells and has advocated that areas where growths have been surgically removed be treated with a chelidonium preparation. Some internal remedies have been documented as well, such as those for gallbladder infections and stones; however, Russian physicians warn these remedies should only be attempted under medical supervision.[91]

In Britain and Ireland, twenty-first-century folk practitioners were found to have a range of applications for *Chelidonium* including as an astringent for removing wrinkles and freckles, as an acrid spring purgative, a kidney stimulant, and for the treatment of cancer of the liver.[92]

As late as the 1950s, in Portugal the herb was still employed in official medicine. In Czechoslovakia it was used as a laxative and diuretic.[93]

CHELIDONIUM MAJUS IN EUROPEAN HERBALISM IN THE EARLY TWENTIETH CENTURY: In Russia chelidonium is called chistotel, which translates to "body-cleanser." The plant is the subject of a traditional folktale in which the twelfth-century princess Natasha is punished with a terrible rash for being part of an adulterous plot. She's healed only after she accidentally brushes up against a chistotel plant she encounters in the forest.[94] Soviet folk healers deployed this plant, mostly the juice extracted from the roots, against diseases of the liver and the bile tract, jaundice, gout, scrofula, ulcers, wounds, and skin diseases such as carcinomas and psoriasis. The juice is useful for removing warts, papillomas, genital warts, and milker's nodules (a condition caused by milking infected cows).[95]

Celandine is one of the main plants depicted in a late-medieval Polish carving that decorates St. Mary's Basilica in Kraków. The detailed relief is a source of information depicting plants that flourished in the region at that time. In the final panel of the series, Christ the gardener is shown with spade in hand, surrounded by lily of the valley, dead nettle, and celandine. Today, as it was in the Middle Ages, celandine is found growing wild all over Poland. Both the Poles and Slovaks use a traditional method for removing warts by directly squeezing the herb's intense yellow latex onto the blemish. In addition Slovaks put fresh leaves on a swollen abdomen, whereas Dalmatians apply the juice to foot ulcers.

At the turn of the twentieth century, celandine, or *Schöllkraut*, grew all along fences and paths in Germany. Folk healers at the time relied widely on this plant, especially its fresh juice, as an excellent way of stimulating the metabolism. It was also, according to one researcher, similar to morphine, reducing pain by producing localized insensitivity. Other treatments targeted liver congestion, biliary disorders, skin conditions, menstrual and hemorrhoidal complaints, swellings, and hardening of the abdominal organs. Additionally the herb was a "particularly popular remedy for syphilis in the secondary stage." In ophthalmology it was used for corneal opacities and chronic eyelid inflammation.[96]

CHELIDONIUM MAJUS IN ASHKENAZI HERBALISM IN THE PALE IN THE EARLY TWENTIETH CENTURY:[97] From a 1938 YIVO publication: "Ver es git a lek di milch fun der milchblum, vert mshuge"—a saying from the town of Sonik (present-day Sanok, Poland): "He who licks the milk from the milkflower will go crazy."[98]

Celandine, or *milkhblum* (Yiddish for "milkflower"), was very common in the Pale at the turn of the twentieth century and could be found in shady places, especially in the forest. At that time the plant's toxic constituents were unknown, so warnings of possible harmful effects were not yet officially stated.

In Ritzev juice from the fresh plant was drunk for constipation, and a decoction made from the dried plant was taken for kidney diseases.

For pain and fainting spells in Polona and Tchan, a strongly brewed plant decoction was drunk. It was also used to wash the scalp.

Celandine was the plant most commonly used for treating skin diseases and wounds. As in contemporary Russian practice, the fresh juice of the plant or the root was poured and rubbed on warts, or a plant decoction was used for the same purpose in Polona, Anapol, Litin, Balte, Lubni, Romen, and Yelisavetgrod.

The same preparation was a remedy for wounds in Yelisavetgrod, Letichev, and Zvenigorodka.

In Broslev the fresh or steamed plant was applied to abscesses and the root rubbed on wounds caused by venereal diseases, which are not specified in the source but echo the German preparation of the same period for syphilis.

In Romen, Lubni, Kiev, Anapol, Polona, Bohslov, Balte, and Monaster-ishtche, the juice or a decoction of the plant was rubbed on locally or a bath was made with a decoction of the plant to heal skin disorders such as itching, eczema, herpes, scrofula, and rash.

Celandine flowers and leaves were used to treat liver diseases in Shvartz-Timeh.

In general in the region, *Chelidonium* was used for diseases of the eyes, as an external and as an internal remedy to prevent leucoma (a white opacity in the cornea of the eye) and the formation of white spots on the cornea.[99]

5
CICHORIUM INTYBUS

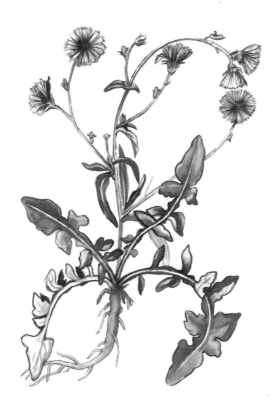

FAMILY: Asteraceae

COMMON ENGLISH NAMES: chicory, succory, wild succory

YIDDISH: צ", צ-קָריע, חילדע

HEBREW: עלש צ-קוריא

UKRAINIAN: Цикорій дикий, Петрові батоги, Петрів батіг, Петрів батіжок, довгий батіг

GERMAN: Wegwart, Gemeine Wegwarte, Zichorie

POLISH: Cykoria podróżnik, podróżnik błękitny

RUSSIAN: Цикорий обыкновенный

LITHUANIAN: Paprastoji trūkažolė

DESCRIPTION AND LOCATION: Perennial native to western Asia, North Africa, and Europe. Its stem can reach two to three feet high with a general appearance of stiff angularity because its branches, while numerous, tend to be spreading, grow at long lengths from the stems, and have few leaves of any size to cover them. Lower leaves, while similar in form to the dandelion's, are large and covered with hairs. Upper leaves are much smaller and less divided than the lower and clasp the stem at their base. Light blue flowers are numerous, generally in clusters of two or three, and bloom from July to September. These open and close with a clocklike regularity that fluctuates with the latitude where the plant grows. Its taproot, similar to the dandelion's *(Taraxacum vulgare)*, is light yellow outside, white inside. The entire plant, including the root, contains a bitter milky latex.[100]

***CICHORIUM INTYBUS* EARLY REMEDIES:** The healing herb chicory has been known since the earliest recorded human history. Homer, who scholars believe lived eight hundred years prior to the Common Era, was known for his description of ancient Egypt, the land famous for its medicinal herbs; among the plants most admired by the Egyptians was chicory.

By the first century of the Common Era, the Greek physician and botanist Dioscorides had included chicory in his writings on medicinal plants; he distinguished two types, wild and cultivated. The former he designated as the more wholesome of the two. He further described the plants as having astringent and cooling properties and that they "comfort a weak stomach and heartburn when eaten." He also recommended that they be made into a plaster with barley groats, or be taken by themselves for the benefit of those with heart ailments, or for treating the skin infection known as erysipelas. Chicory was also considered useful for gout or eye inflammations. Scorpion stings, common in ancient Greece, were treated with the entire plant including the root, and the juice of the plant was smeared with white lead and vinegar on inflamed skin conditions.[101]

British herbalist Maude Grieve vacillates on the origin of chicory's name. She first postulated that one of its titles, succory, may have come from the Latin *succurrere*, "to run under," because of the depths the herb's roots reach. Its true origin, however, may come from a corruption of the ancient Egyptian word for the plant. Ancient Arabic physicians referred to the plant as *chicourey*.[102]

The physician Tobias ha-Kohen, in his text *Ma'aseh Toviyah* ("Work of Tobias"), wrote in Hebrew with many loan words mixed in. He referred to the plant "*tzikoria*," a cognate for *cicoria*, the Italian word for chicory, and recommended its use mainly for women's health and for digestive concerns, especially with regard to children.[103]

Intybus, the specific name for the plant, according to Grieve, is another modification of a word that also finds its origins in the East: *hendibeh* (Arabic). The physician Maimonides wrote on the origins of *intybus* as well and observed that its name originated as the Greek word *antubiya*; modern scholars believe that, like *chicory*, the specific also derives from ancient Egyptian.[104]

Some biblical scholars believe chicory is one of the "bitter herbs," or "maror," eaten by Jews on the festival of Passover, since the plant was believed to have been widely distributed and common in Egypt and southwestern Asia.[105] But botanists regard chicory as native to India and have expressed doubt as to whether it would have been introduced into Egypt and Palestine at the time of Moses (in the middle of the second millennium BCE), or that trade in chicory would have been established at that time because it was not a plant that would have survived the journey in a fresh state.[106]

The Romans ate chicory as a vegetable or in salads.[107]

Sixteenth-century herbalists believed its leaves, when crushed and used as a poultice, were helpful for swellings and inflammations, including irritated eyes. And if boiled and eaten in a broth, the plant was able to cool down hot, weak digestive systems.[108]

The Cherokee know chicory's root as a nervine tonic.[109]

***CICHORIUM INTYBUS* CONTEMPORARY ACTIONS:** tonic, bitter, appetite stimulant, hepatic, antioxidant

CICHORIUM INTYBUS **CONTEMPORARY MEDICINAL PARTS:** root

CICHORIUM INTYBUS **IN CONTEMPORARY HERBALISM:** Today chicory is no longer the revered medicine it was in times past. In most of Europe and the United States, only chicory's root is considered of value; when roasted, it contributes to the flavor of coffee. Some contemporary North American herbalists commonly recommend root preparations to stimulate the appetite and digestion and to treat liver disorders and gallstones.[110] In TCM, however, the plant is known to enhance fire or yang characteristics in healing formulations.[111]

In Germany chicory has been accepted into official medicine as a treatment for loss of appetite and dyspepsia.[112] One contemporary German herbalist mentions in passing chicory's root can be added to a tea for gallbladder health, yet describes the plant as "enjoying the sides of dusty streets heavy with traffic."[113] While it might seem strange to say, the plants we need most are the ones that grow closest to us, or even the plants we happen to notice out of the corner of our eye. In my own experience lemon balm, cleavers, horsetail, and violet are among the plants that sprung up spontaneously around my house. I didn't plant them, yet I find I need them more often than I would have anticipated. Wherever I go, I try to notice what plants are present and where they are growing because it says a lot about the people who spend time there. In the case of chicory growing so profusely where people travel, it could be inferred that most of those who speed through the area could probably benefit from the herb's medicine.

In the text *Principles and Practice of Phytotherapy,* the authors recommend cooling bitters, like Taraxacum, Gentiana, and Cichorium and Erythraea for a gentle reduction in temperature during a fever, and they add that these bitters have the extra advantage of stimulating the digestive system to help counter fermentation or infection in the gut that may have arisen due to the body's preoccupation with combatting a pathogen.[114]

Scientific studies show chicory's effect on cholesterol, and in one experiment the herb was shown to be antioxidant.[115]

CICHORIUM INTYBUS **IN EUROPEAN HERBALISM IN THE EARLY TWENTIETH CENTURY:** By the early 1900s chicory was still widely used and much cultivated on the Continent, especially for its large and fleshy root. In the 1930s it was roasted, ground, and mixed with coffee. In the twenty-first century in the

United States, this recipe is still a popular beverage, especially in New Orleans, where it's one of the city's most touted nonalcoholic choices.

Europeans of the early twentieth century foraged the plant's fresh bitter root for its medicinal actions. Its milky juice provided a mild laxative, or aperient effect, and because it was slightly sedative, it was found to be helpful for those troubled with "bilious torpor." It was also suitable for those who suffered from "pulmonary consumption." Other health issues of the era treated with chicory included jaundice, enlarged liver, gout, and skin eruptions connected with rheumatism; a decoction of the fresh plant was recommended for urinary tract "gravel." And because it's nonirritating, it was considered an excellent laxative for children.[116]

In Germany the plant served as a stomach remedy, and a tonic of the root, flower, and fruit was formulated for a variety of illnesses including catarrh, hypochondria, hysteria, jaundice, rabies, scurvy, and blood in urine, in addition to strengthening gastric weakness. In Swabia the plant was regarded as enchanted: the blue flowers were associated with evil while the white were thought to be good. In Franconia chicory protected against all kinds of magic; and in Swabia the root was believed to have the strength to remove thorns and splinters and other wayward objects from the flesh—but also keep the wearer of the plant safe from witches and immune to swords and skewers. In western Bohemia chicory was associated with Christianity. If one approached the plant in the correct manner, recited a specific prayer, then pulled the root, washed it with running water, put it in a silk bag, and, finally, carried it with them, they would be certain to find hidden treasures and all barriers would be removed for them.[117]

As healthful as this plant could be, it was also considered to be harmful if taken too regularly, possibly causing digestive issues in overzealous admirers.[118]

Poles steeped its roots in spirytus, a high-alcohol grain beverage, along with the leaves and roots of anise. This infusion was used as a remedy for cholera and other abdominal pain. Additionally the mountain people of Poland used the roots to bathe children suffering from tuberculosis.[119]

Slovakian girls wore the plant under the sole of their right boot, possibly to encourage male admirers. In more medicinal realms Slovaks made a decoction of the flowers that they used to wash inflamed eyelids. It was also drunk in small portions for excessive menstrual flow; however, women were cautioned not to enjoy too much of this liquid or their menses would be curtailed for possibly up to three years. In addition chicory flowers were placed on warts between fingers to "drive them away." Besides being used to bathe children with a fever, as in German lands, the plant was also often used in magic medicine.[120]

In Dalmatia chicory was brewed in a decoction to remedy hemorrhoids, clear the head, cleanse the blood, treat fever, and help those with blood in their urine.[121]

Formerly, in Russia, decoctions and root extracts were generally used as bitters. In folk medicine the plant was a popular treatment for liver diseases, especially jaundice and cirrhosis, tumors of the spleen and stomach, intestinal disorders, overall weakness, and eczema. It was also recommended for diabetics and was employed as an anthelmintic in veterinary medicine.[122]

***CICHORIUM INTYBUS* IN ASHKENAZI HERBALISM IN THE PALE IN THE EARLY TWENTIETH CENTURY:**[123] As in contemporary Germany, in the Pale chicory was commonly found growing on rubbish heaps and along highways. In folk medicine of the region, chicory was mainly sought for the relief of stomach and intestinal ailments. The herb's roots, or sometimes the whole plant, were dug up for this purpose.

In little towns such as Anapol and Lachovitz, both adults and children who suffered from diarrhea drank a decoction made with one teaspoon of the powdered dried root to one glass of boiling water. Children were instructed to take one teaspoon three to four times a day, while adults took one tablespoon at the same frequency. In these two towns this same preparation was given for relief from "catarrh of the stomach."

In Olt-Kosntin a decocted ratio of three plants to one glass of water was taken as a vermifuge; this remedy promised intestinal parasites would pass after twenty-four hours.

In the town of Broslev a combined decoction of chicory, sweet flag (*Acorus calamus*), and wormwood (*Artemisia absinthium*) was given by folk healers to treat hemorrhoids.

Other bodily ailments, apart from those directly affecting digestion, were also helped by the herb in the towns and villages of the Pale. For example, in the western Ukrainian towns of Zaslov and Polona folk healers gave a decoction made from the plant's stem as a mouthwash to relieve toothache.

In Ulanov a decoction was drunk to remedy lung ailments including shortness of breath.

This same decoction was drunk for rheumatism and colds in Ladizhin.

In Kiev chicory was used to treat bites from "mad dogs," a remedy similar to one known in Germany.

Chicory also was valued for women's health in the Pale. In Litin a midwife advised a root decoction or tincture was to be taken on an empty stomach by women to stop menstrual bleeding, which very much echoed chicory's application in Slovakia. Litin midwives also recommended a bath with chicory for (unspecified) gynecological disease.

In nearby Khmelnik in the Vinnitsa region, a decoction of the entire herb was given to women during delivery to accelerate the passing of the placenta.

An interesting comparison can be seen with the use of chicory in the Bessarabian town of Birzula, where a healer prepared a decoction of chicory to wash wounds and abscesses or soaked a compress with the liquid to treat similar conditions. Two hundred years earlier, in the *Ma'aseh Toviyah*, there can be found a reference to the use of chicory in a compress to treat skin irritations.[124]

While reliance on chicory as a remedy appears common in the towns and villages of Eastern Europe, it is especially worth noting that this herb was often looked to for treating children's ailments in those communities. In the early eighteenth century, the university-trained physician Tobias ha-Kohen wrote that children could safely take this herb for several health concerns, including stomach upset and constipation.[125] Two hundred years later the use of chicory for the restoration of children's health can be seen in Ritzev, where youngsters were treated for insomnia by bathing them in a decoction of the plant. The same type of bath was a remedy in Litin to calm children who cried inconsolably. In Broslev a similar formula was used for infants who suffered from bloody diarrhea. In Monasterishtche and further north and west in the larger town of Barditchev, chicory was a nourishing drink for marasmic, or severely malnourished, children.

In the Podolia region chicory was often used as a laxative. In Derazhnia, a town close to Letichev, Rose Psotta describes a typical daily family meal in her memoir as "cereal made of barley grits, cocoa or hot chicory and milk."[126]

Folk veterinary medicine in the Pale also relied heavily on the plant for farm animal health. In Monasterishtche, Bohslov, and Korsn, chicory as feed was given to increase lactation in cattle; in Khmelnik it helped with the passing of the cow's placenta during delivery.

6

CYNOGLOSSUM OFFICINALE

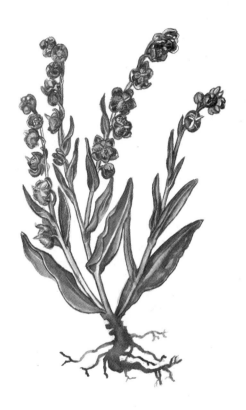

FAMILY: Boraginaceae

COMMON ENGLISH NAMES: houndstongue, houndstooth, dog's tongue, gypsy flower, rats and mice, dog-bur, sheeplice, woolmat

YIDDISH: שוואַרצוואַרצל

HEBREW: לשון כלב

UKRAINIAN: Чорнокорінь лікарський, чорнокорінь, воловий язик, совачий язик, реп'яшник, язичник, лишайник, майник, золотник, гадючий бур'ян, бородавник, білий корінь, бідник, ранненик, натягач, медвеже вушко, живокість, заложник, сіре зілля, гав'язь

GERMAN: Gewöhnliche Hundszunge

POLISH: Ostrzeń pospolity, ostrzeń purpurowy, psi język

RUSSIAN: Чернокорень аптечный, чернокорень лекарственный

LITHUANIAN: Vaistinė šunlielė

DESCRIPTION AND LOCATION: Biennial that produces an erect stem that can reach one to three feet high and bears alternating lance-shaped—like a dog's tongue—leaves covered with down that are directly attached to the stem. Flowers are reddish-purple and funnel-shaped, grow in curling clusters, or racemes, and bloom from May to September. Houndstongue is found in waste areas, in sandy, rocky soil, and along roadsides. In North America it grows throughout the Great Plains, from Montana to Kansas. When bruised, the plant emits an unpleasant odor described as "mouse-like."[127]

CYNOGLOSSUM OFFICINALE **EARLY REMEDIES:** Houndstongue is unique among the plants identified as medicinal in the Pale because it was not included in the classic Greek sources where many medicinal plants are documented. Could this be interpreted as *Cynoglossum officinale* being an Indigenous remedy or possibly one that was adopted from sources other than the ancients? In any event, one of the earliest written acknowledgments of the plant's medicinal qualities can be found in English botanist John Gerard's text, which advises readers to put the herb's leaves on the bottoms of the feet, presumably within a shoe, to "tye the tongues of Houndes so that they shall not bark at you." The plant was also applied as an ointment or decoction, both of which were generally regarded as a remedy for rabies.[128]

By the time English botanist and physician Nicholas Culpeper set down his medical expertise in the seventeenth century, the root was used for coughs, colds in the head, and shortness of breath. The leaves were a cure for dysentery. Other preparations were said to reduce hair loss and soothe scalds and hemorrhoids.[129]

Paracelsus reminded his readers that "many herbs and roots got their names, not from any one inborn virtue and faculty, but from their figure, form, and appearance," and among these he included *Cynoglossum*.[130]

CYNOGLOSSUM OFFICINALE CONTEMPORARY ACTIONS: astringent

CYNOGLOSSUM OFFICINALE CONTEMPORARY MEDICINAL PARTS: aerial and root

CYNOGLOSSUM OFFICINALE IN CONTEMPORARY HERBALISM: Internally the herb's use has been primarily to clear up diarrhea, and topically for burns, bruises, and hard-to-heal wounds. The crushed plant has also been applied to treat insect bites. While rarely listed in contemporary western herbals, when it is, houndstongue's medicinal qualities are not highly praised. The plant is considered toxic, and if used internally at all, herbalists caution, this should be done so with the utmost care.[131]

A related plant, the Pacific hound's tongue (*Adelinia grande*, previously known as *Cynoglossum grande*), grows along the central and northern coastal mountain ranges of western North America from California to British Columbia. Indigenous peoples have used its root in a tea to treat gonorrhea and other sexually transmitted diseases. This relative is also considered toxic and internal use should be avoided.[132]

In Ireland preparations of the cultivated plant have been valued as a remedy for coughs and its heated leaves as a hot dressing for burns.[133]

CYNOGLOSSUM OFFICINALE IN HERBALISM IN THE EARLY TWENTIETH CENTURY: While not a European source strictly speaking, houndstongue was regarded by the Eclectic school of American herbalism—which incorporated Native American plants and applications into a European herbal tradition—as an anodyne, demulcent, and astringent; the Eclectics further noted that the plant was taken internally as a remedy for coughs, catarrhs, hemoptysis, diarrhea, and dysentery. Externally they found it to be a healing poultice for scrofulous tumors, burns, goiter, skin wounds, or inflammations. The plant proved helpful for the immediate relief of pain from the soreness caused by irritated, bruised, or chafed areas, especially from prolonged use of the feet. And for ecchymosis (a discoloration of the skin resulting from bleeding underneath, typically caused by bruising), the tincture was known to reduce swelling and discoloration. Almost as an afterthought the Eclectics also provided the vague caution: "Paralyzing effects are said to be produced by it in the vertebrate animals."[134]

Meanwhile, in the British Isles of the early twentieth century, the plant was still often used internally and externally to relieve hemorrhoids and was thought to be soothing to the digestive organs.[135]

In the early years of the twentieth century in Ireland, where houndstongue commonly grows, one folk medicinal topical use was recorded where juice of a wild specimen was rubbed on irritations known as felons.[136]

In Russian folk medicine, preparations of houndstongue were taken internally to soothe pain, cramping, and coughs, and applied externally for boils, burns, and snakebites. In some parts of Russia, the juice and roots were also used as an insecticide and rodent repellent.[137]

CYNOGLOSSUM OFFICINALE IN ASHKENAZI HERBALISM IN THE PALE IN THE EARLY TWENTIETH CENTURY:[138] By the middle of the twentieth century houndstongue's shortcomings had been identified, and consequently use of its medicine internally was rendered unacceptable. But when the Soviets conducted their ethnobotanical surveys between the world wars, houndstongue was still a viable folk remedy. In the Pale the plant grew in and around the small towns and along the highways and slopes that connected them. While most of the folk healers in the towns and villages must have intuited the plant's medicine was best drawn upon topically, a few traditional practitioners at the time must have considered the plant safe to ingest. Also of note is the plant's application in gynecological treatments.

In Ladizhin a bath made with the dried leaf and root decoction was given to those suffering from colds or rheumatism, and in Yekaterinoslav this same bath was also taken for rheumatic pain.

A root decoction was used to mend bone fractures in Kiev, possibly as a substitute for comfrey (*Symphytum officinale*).

Folk healers in Slovita dried and then powdered the root to sprinkle on wounds, or else fresh leaves or leaves steamed in water were applied to wounds.

Ground fresh roots and leaves were poulticed for festering wounds in Korosten and Slovita.

In Zvenigorodka a dried root tincture was poured drop by drop on wounds.

Cherkoss folk practitioners decocted the whole plant and washed wounds caused by eczema, while in Litin the same brew was applied to herpes sores after the blisters had broken.

The fresh plant, including the root, mixed with grease (Ossadcha-Janata does not specify, but it is likely that her generic references to "grease" are to goose, rather than bear, tallow, lard, etc.) then ground was the recipe for a salve folk healers made for rubbing on children and adults suffering from itch in Ladizhin.

In Bohslov the plant's juice was applied to warts to remove them.

Remarkably, in an application that mirrors that of Native Americans, Barditchev folk practitioners made a decoction of the plant that was taken internally as a remedy for venereal diseases.

In Ladizhin midwives prepared poultices made with the plant decoction that were applied topically to stop menstruation. Men in Ladizhin were given an identical poultice to cure hemorrhoids, and the same preparation was a remedy to staunch nosebleeds.

Midwives in Anapol created an infusion of the whole plant, which was taken by women to induce menstruation.

After childbirth a root tincture was given to women in Balte.

Marasmic (emaciated) children in Broslev who were severely malnourished and underweight were both bathed in a decoction of houndstongue and advised to drink a similar formula.

7
DELPHINIUM CONSOLIDA

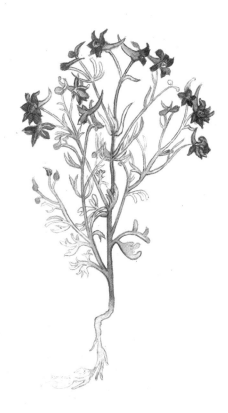

FAMILY: Ranunculaceae

COMMON ENGLISH NAMES: forking larkspur, rocket-larkspur, field larkspur, lark heels (Shakespeare)

YIDDISH: זשיוועקיסט ,ריטערשפּאָרן

HEBREW: דרבנית

UKRAINIAN: Сокирки польові, сокирки, житні сокирки, сокирки синенькі, косарики, косирки, серпоріз, серпики, сенець, синя вода, тоя польова, козельці

GERMAN: Gewöhnliche Feldrittersporn, Acker-Rittersporn, Feldrittersporn

POLISH: Ostróżka, ostróżeczka polna, ostróżka polna

RUSSIAN: Живокость полевая, шпорник, сокирки полевые

DESCRIPTION AND LOCATION: Annual with a slender taproot; upright round stem divides alternately into leafy branches and can reach two to four feet in height. Lower alternate leaves attach to stems with short half-inch stalks, while higher leaves are mainly attached directly to the plant's stem. Clusters of pink, purple, or blue flowers attach to stem on short equal stalks that give way to black flattened seeds that are odorless but toxic. Often grown as an ornamental, *Delphinium consolida* is also found in fecund and dry forests or along rocky slopes. Common in Europe and North America; blooms from June to August.[139] Caution is advised when handling this plant especially with regard to children.[140]

***DELPHINIUM CONSOLIDA* EARLY REMEDIES:** The name Delphinium, from the Latin delphinus (dolphin), comes from the genus's flower buds, which were thought to resemble a dolphin. And despite the fact that its species name refers to the plant's power of consolidating wounds, the ancients disregarded *Delphinium consolida* and instead wrote of a closely related plant, *Delphinium staphisagria*, or stavesacre. Dioscorides knew stavesacre to be a poison, but it was used in his time as an emetic, to rid one of lice, as an expectorant, to "staunch rheumy gums," and to treat oral thrush.[141]

In Renaissance Poland imported *Delphiniums* gave color to formal gardens.[142]

By the seventeenth century Nicholas Culpeper, writing of "Consolida Regalis, Delphinium," also referred to the plant as "Lark heels," the name attributed to Shakespeare, who included it in the lyrics for the introductory song to the play "The Two Noble Kinsmen." Culpeper also noted the plant's abilities to "resist poison" and to "help the bitings of venomous beasts."[143]

***DELPHINIUM CONSOLIDA* CONTEMPORARY ACTIONS:** anthelmintic, purgative

DELPHINIUM CONSOLIDA **CONTEMPORARY MEDICINAL PARTS:** seed

DELPHINIUM CONSOLIDA **IN CONTEMPORARY HERBALISM:** By the late nineteen sixties and early seventies, American herbalists found branching larkspur to be too weak as a medicinal plant, but toxic if large quantities were consumed. At most its seeds were considered a parasiticide for killing head lice or other external vermin.[144]

DELPHINIUM CONSOLIDA **IN EUROPEAN HERBALISM IN THE EARLY TWENTIETH CENTURY:** In 1930s Britain, *Delphinium consolida* was described as identical to stavesacre, in both its medicinal qualities and its toxicity. It was primarily counted on externally to destroy lice and hair nits, and during the First World War, soldiers in the trenches applied it in this way with great success. A tincture made from the seeds and gradually titrated up was also considered beneficial for treating spasmodic asthma and dropsy. Juice pressed from the leaves was thought helpful for treating bleeding hemorrhoids. For children, a jam made from the plant's flowers had been considered "excellent medicine" for cases of extreme vomiting; another preparation of the plant was prescribed to quell colic.

In both the British Isles and North America, branching larkspur was sought for its utility as a blue dye.[145]

At the turn of the twentieth century, Slovakian folk medicine practitioners gave a decoction of branching larkspur for treating those with blood in the urine. Women were given this tea after childbirth to speed the elimination of the afterbirth. Slovaks also burned the dried herb to treat the facial rose, or erysipelas, by fumigation.[146]

In twentieth-century Poland a related species, the *Delphinium elatum*, was still a feature of cottage gardens, and women placed the leaves of branching larkspur beneath bed sheets to discourage fleas. Larkspur root was drunk with milk to strengthen weak hearts.[147] In Russian folk medicine the plant's flowers were employed as an anthelmintic and diuretic.[148]

DELPHINIUM CONSOLIDA **IN ASHKENAZI HERBALISM IN THE PALE IN THE EARLY TWENTIETH CENTURY:[149]** Branching larkspur was a common weed in the Pale between the wars and could be found growing in fields, on farmland, and along highways. It was widely used in the folk medicine of Eastern Europe.

In Ladizhin folk healers made a decoction of flowers or of the whole plant as a cordial that was given as a diuretic.

The same preparation was given for the treatment of kidney diseases in Birzula.

In Cherkoss folk healers relied on *Delphinium consolida* to treat diarrhea, bloody diarrhea, and dysentery.

In Korsn it was offered for stomach pain.

Healers in Romen and Anapol gave those suffering from constipation the same remedy.

A similar decoction was often given to women to stop bleeding or to induce menstruation or to expel the placenta in Polona, Ritzev, Litin, Ulanov, Kolenivka, Korosten, Makhnivke, Birzula, Kanev, Cherkoss, Bohslov, Zvenigorodka, Lyubashivka, Savran, Balte, Bazilia, Monasterishtche, and Broslev. This placental use is parallel to that of the Slovaks of the same era, mentioned earlier.

In Kresilev a tincture or decoction of dried flowers was a remedy for toothache.

A decoction made of the roots, cut into pieces and mixed with *Menyanthes trifoliata* (bogbean or buckbean) and birch and pine buds, was used for tuberculosis in Kiev. Additionally a root decoction of the plant alone was applied locally in the form of compresses and poultices to swellings.

In folk veterinary medicine an aqueous solution of the plant or flowers served as a diuretic in Romen, Shvartz-Timeh, and Ladizhin.

In Ritzev, Barditchev, Olt-Kosntin, Vinitza, Litin, Korosten, and Makhnivke the same water-based solution was used when cows could not expel the placenta after calving.

In Romen and Hadyitsh, it was given to animals as an astringent to treat diarrhea.

The plant's flowers were also utilized as a blue dye for cloth; the same practice is noted in both Britain and North America.

8

EQUISETUM ARVENSE

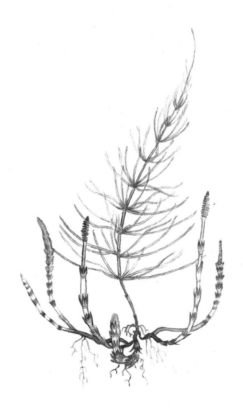

FAMILY: Equisetaceae

COMMON ENGLISH NAMES: field horsetail, horsetail rush, horsetail grass, shave grass, bottle-brush, paddock-pipes, Dutch rushes, pewterwort

YIDDISH: שלייפֿגראָז, קייטלדרות

HEBREW: שבטכט

UKRAINIAN: Сосонка польова, хвощ польовий, сосонка, полевий хвощ, хвощ, хвищ, майові губкі - весняні спороносні гони

GERMAN: Schachtelhalm, Zinnkraut, Zinngras, Katzenwedel, Pferdeschwanz, Schaftheu, Pfannebutzer, Scheuerkraut

POLISH: Ziela skrzypu, skrzyp polny

RUSSIAN: Хвощ полевой, толкачик

LITHUANIAN: Dirvinis asiūklis

DESCRIPTION AND LOCATION: Nonflowering perennial common in moist loam or sandy soil along roadsides, excavated areas, and gardens all over North America and Eurasia. A stringlike root is divided by nodes from which roots grow. From these nodes arise numerous hollow stems, of which there are two types. The first is fertile and can grow from four to seven inches, eventually bearing a cone-like top that holds the plant's spores. After this short-lived stem dies back, a green, hollow, sterile stem appears, reaching up to eighteen inches in height with whorls of short branched segments growing from each of its nodes and tapering in size and length as they reach the top of the stem.[150] In this way the plant resembles a horse's tail.

***EQUISETUM ARVENSE* EARLY REMEDIES:** Ancestors of the field horsetail found in the fossil record of common coal reveal a plant that flourished around 370 million years ago and attained heights of one hundred feet. The only ostensible difference between today's plant and those behemoths of the Carboniferous age is their relative size.[151]

Two thousand years ago, when Dioscorides wrote of the genus in addressing *Equisetum silvaticum*, he set down its medicinal qualities as astringent, its juice's ability to staunch nosebleeds, and its efficacy against dysentery. Ground up and plastered on, it was able to seal bleeding wounds; the roots, when combined with the rest of the plant, soothed coughs and helped those with the shortness of breath lying prone can cause. He also noted its ability to mend breaks in the intestines, ruptured bladders, and intestinal hernias when drunk as a water solution.[152]

A millennium and a half later, John Gerard related that the plant was great for scouring pewter and wooden kitchen utensils, and it had consequently been given the title *pewterwort*. Fast-forward a few hundred years and the dairymaids of the northern counties of England were using the plant for scrubbing the milk pails of their trade. Even today it is still said that powdered horsetail ash mixed with water is the best silver cleaner.[153]

Nicholas Culpeper chronicled horsetail's many medicinal virtues, reiterating its powerful ability to stop bleeding both internally and externally, as well as its capacity to heal internal ulcers. In addition he wrote that it soldered together fresh wounds and ruptures in children. For the urinary tract it was helpful for reducing stone and strangury. As a drink it was infused in distilled water to strengthen the intestines, ease coughs, and soothe skin irritations and inflammations.[154]

Seventeenth-century Polish botanist Simon Syreniusz recommended preparing the herb with wine for healing dysentery and bloody lungs. He also suggested placing horsetail in a bath, a compress, or a rub to heal wounds caused by duels. The dried plant was used as a powder mixed with water to treat ulcers of the liver and uterus and taken with wine it healed intestinal wounds and stomach ulcers.[155]

Mid-nineteenth-century Bavarian priest Sebastian Kneipp recommended the plant for internal bleeding and bloody vomit. To strengthen and improve the appetite of their prized horses, Roma living in Poland added the plant to their feed.[156]

Native peoples in North America made a tea from the stem as a diuretic, a kidney tonic, and a laxative. Topically they applied it as a poultice to astringe underarm and groin irritations. The stems were also powdered and sprinkled in footwear to prevent cramping during long distance travel or burned to ash to heal sore mouths or wash itching or open sores.[157]

EQUISETUM ARVENSE **CONTEMPORARY ACTIONS:** diuretic, hemostatic, vulnerary, mineralizer, astringent, anti-inflammatory, coagulant

EQUISETUM ARVENSE **CONTEMPORARY MEDICINAL PARTS:** aboveground parts, harvested in summer

EQUISETUM ARVENSE **IN CONTEMPORARY HERBALISM:** Today herbalists find the plant's high mineral content to be most beneficial for skin, hair, and bone health.[158] Because silica, one of its chief constituents, is soluble in water, it's easily transported throughout the body. Teas made from horsetail take advantage of this virtue and can strengthen body tissues with elasticity, without making them brittle.[159] In some cases this preparation can rebuild joints and other connective tissues. The plant has also been praised for treating mild cases of tuberculosis because its silicic acid constituent has been said to stabilize scar tissue.[160]

Because it promotes blood coagulation, the juice of horsetail has been found beneficial for treating anemia caused by internal bleeding from conditions such as stomach ulcers. A horsetail tea has also been known to help with leg ulcers, urinary tract issues, and water retention and to promote gynecological health in cases of excessive menstrual flow and leucorrhea. Externally, wounds, skin, mouth and gum inflammations can be washed with the infusion.[161]

By the late twentieth century, incontinence and bed-wetting in children have been added to the list of urinary ailments horsetail can address with its gentle diuretic actions. It is also considered a specific for benign enlargement of the prostate gland in men. In some cases chilblains and rheumatism complaints have been noted to lessen from use of this herb.[162] Horsetail is also useful in teas for cystitis and other bladder issues.[163]

British medical herbalists consider the herb one of several possible plants able to help replace potassium lost through the use of modern diuretic prescription drugs.[164]

In Germany the plant has been approved for treatment of edema and as a part of an antiseptic irrigation therapy for urinary tract illnesses.[165]

Equisetum arvense, found throughout Russia, has been used in folk medicine for hundreds of years. The young green shoots or stems are drunk as a tea for a fast and long-lasting diuretic effect by those with heart trouble and kidney disease. The plant is also seen as a healing agent for inflammatory diseases of the urinary tract, for treating atherosclerosis that affects the blood vessels of the heart and brain, and for slow-healing ulcers, purulent wounds, and furuncles. For mucus membranes of the mouth or eyes, a cold decoction is used as either a gargle or as a conjunctivitis wash for the eyes. For oily skin, cool compresses with the decocted plant are found to be helpful. As a coagulant, preparations of the plant are beneficial for decreasing excessive menstrual and hemorrhoidal bleeding. In a parallel remedy to one offered by American herbalists, fresh horsetail juice has been given to those suffering from tuberculosis complicated by anemia resulting from bleeding stomach ulcers. Based on the known chemical and biological properties of *Equisetum arvense*, Russian folk herbalists have relied on this herb for generations, if not intentionally then intuitively, to stimulate the immune system.[166]

Nine different types of horsetail grow in Poland. Folk healers there seek out the plant to make a decoction for treating rheumatism, neuralgia, or excessive perspiration. Another Polish folk recipe for treating oily skin includes a combination of burdock root, dried nettle leaves, and dried horsetail, which are decocted for a topical rinse. To rinse oily hair, a cleansing wash combines dried, powdered horsetail, burdock root, chamomile, soapwort, and nettle added to boiling water and then cooled before use.[167]

All herbalists caution that excessive consumption of horsetail may lead to a thiamine deficiency, and the powdered herb is not recommended for children.

EQUISETUM ARVENSE IN EUROPEAN HERBALISM IN THE EARLY TWENTIETH CENTURY: In the British Isles, only horsetail's barren stems were used in their entirety, and they were thought to be most effective when fresh. Mainly sought for its diuretic and astringent properties, horsetail was helpful for treating cases of dropsy, urinary gravel, kidney infections, and the spitting of blood.

A strong decoction of the plant acted as an emmenagogue; its cooling and astringent characteristics made it helpful for staunching hemorrhages and for healing cystic ulcerations and ulcers in the urinary passages. A decoction applied externally stopped bleeding wounds and accelerated healing. This same preparation was also used to reduce the swelling of eyelids. In the early twentieth century, English country people were still gathering the herb to stop nosebleeds, as Culpeper had advised centuries prior. The ashes from the burnt plant were considered valuable in regulating acidity of the stomach and for dyspepsia.[168]

In Switzerland horsetail was recommended as a washing and bathing fluid for festering ulcers, poorly healing wounds, and skin rashes, as well as a tea or decoction taken internally for all disorders of the urinary tract.[169] In Russian folk medicine, preparations made from horsetail were beneficial for hemostasis and against gout, liver diseases, and tuberculosis. Extracts and tinctures from horsetail were given as diuretics, for flushing out edemas, for treating urinary tract inflammation, and to staunch hemorrhoidal bleeding and menorrhagia. Some cautioned that as a diuretic, horsetail could irritate the kidneys, and hence it was less preferred than the alternative treatment of uva ursi.[170]

EQUISETUM ARVENSE IN ASHKENAZI HERBALISM IN THE PALE IN THE EARLY TWENTIETH CENTURY:[171] Horsetail was commonly found growing in the fields, meadows, glades, and forests of the Pale between the world wars.

In the Podolia region *Equisetum arvense* was used to promote urination.[172]

In Shvartz-Timeh, Uman, and Birzula a decoction of horsetail was used to treat kidney diseases.

In Shvartz-Timeh it was also given as a diuretic.

For tuberculosis, head colds, and cough, healers in Kiev, Anapol, Bohslov, and Zvenigorodka gave their patients a decoction of the plant.

The same decoction was prescribed for shortness of breath in Zhitomir and for gout in Shvartz-Timeh; and for those who suffered from catarrh of the stomach, the folk practitioners in Broslev and Ladizhin offered them the same strong brew.

Folk healers washed wounds with an infusion of the plant in Ritzev to protect them from infections.

In Ladizhin a compress soaked with the decocted plant treated eczema.

In Kharkov eczema-infected areas were exposed to a steaming plant decoction while the patient was simultaneously given a strongly brewed combination of horsetail with several other (unspecified) herbs to drink.

Healers in Shvartz-Timeh, Uman, and Zvenigorodka, in an identical treatment to that found in Poland, gave those suffering from rheumatism and rheumatic pain a steam foot bath to treat feet and other affected parts of the body.

To stop excessive menstrual bleeding, midwives in Monasterishtche and Kanev gave women the plant decoction to drink. To induce menstruation, the same drink was given in Monasterishtche.

Midwives in Ulanov and Kolenivka also relied on this remedy to stop hemorrhaging during childbirth.

In Broslev midwives turned to the same brew for (unspecified) diseases of the uterus, a treatment similar to one attested in seventeenth-century Poland for ulcers of that organ.

In Khmelnik and Polona the decoction was also a well-known styptic for staunching a nosebleed or bleeding in the throat.

In Barditchev horsetail was a remedy against hemorrhoids, mirroring a treatment noted in Russian folk medicine.

In Letichev folk veterinary medicine sought the plant for the treatment of bloody urine in cattle.

9
FILIPENDULA HEXAPETALA

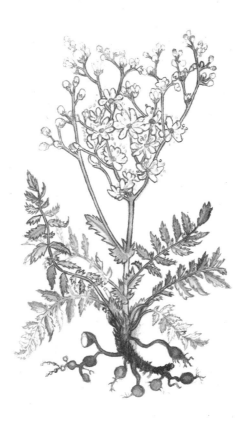

NOTE: According to the September 1967 issue of the *American Journal of Botany*, the accepted binomial for dropwort is *Filipendula vulgaris Moench.* Synonyms for this species include *Filipendula hexapetala*, which was the Latin name known for the plant commonly found in Eastern European folk medicine between the world wars and which is the focus of this profile. Maude Grieve includes the plant in *A Modern Herbal* under the entry for meadowsweet, a closely related plant, and refers to dropwort as *"Spiraea Filipendula."*

FAMILY: Rosaceae

COMMON ENGLISH NAMES: dropwort or fern-leaf dropwort

YIDDISH: שפּירקוסט

UKRAINIAN: Гадючник, лабазник шестипелюстковий, балабани, балабан, балабанчики, балабанчик, балабон, балабони, балабончики, талабан, бобони, горішок, золотник, стожильник, майській бальзан, ранник, починочки, горілочки, кашка-квіти, буранчики, земляне серце, порушник, формулівка

POLISH: Wiezówka błotna, tawula błotna, wiązówka, wiązówka bulwkowata

GERMAN: Mädesüß

RUSSIAN: Лабазнык шестилипестный, таболга шестилепестная

DESCRIPTION AND LOCATION: Perennial that grows in dry pasturelands across much of northern Eurasia. When in flower, dropwort can reach a foot in height. A short rhizome produces many nodules, or knots, and from these grow rootlets.

Leaves, like those of ferns, are pinnate, meaning many leaflets grow opposite each other on either side of a central stem. Before opening, buds are tinged pink externally, but once in bloom they are white and grow in erect crowded clusters. What distinguishes dropwort from its close relative meadowsweet are its pink buds, its scentless white flowers, and its elegantly cut leaves. Blooms in June and July.[173]

FILIPENDULA HEXAPETALA **EARLY REMEDIES:** For the ancient Greeks, dropwort (first known as *Spiraea filipendula* and later classified as *Filipendula hexapetala*) was not as popular a medicinal herb as others of the era. Dioscorides described its above-ground parts as a gynecological medicine that cleared the afterbirth; the root was drunk with wine to treat strangury.[174] Subsequently Galen added dropwort's cooling properties' positive effect on the stomach but warned that if the plant had not been collected on an exact specified calendar day, sometime around the summer solstice, its flowers were not to be trusted.[175]

By the time botanist John Gerard wrote in the early seventeenth century, things were getting a little complicated. The scented meadowsweet, that very close relative of dropwort, had come into broader usage in western Europe, and many herbalists, including Gerard and Culpeper, ardently praised meadowsweet's virtues, seemingly to leave dropwort by the wayside. Why was this? Could it have been that dropwort grew mainly in the east and meadowsweet was more ubiquitous in northwestern Europe? In western Europe meadowsweet met with such immediate success that it was prescribed for measles, smallpox, dysentery, malignant fevers, diarrhea, the spitting up of blood, and hemorrhoids.[176] But what was the difference between meadowsweet and dropwort aside from their physical distinctions? Medicinally, as herbalists have pointed out, the two plants' actions are equivalent.[177] Therefore, in order to allow them to retain their individual identities, each will be mentioned here by name as appropriate.

FILIPENDULA HEXAPETALA (DROPWORT) AND *FILIPENDULA ULMARIA* (MEADOWSWEET) CONTEMPORARY ACTIONS: antirheumatic, anti-inflammatory, carminative, antacid, antiemetic, astringent

FILIPENDULA HEXAPETALA CONTEMPORARY MEDICINAL PARTS: aerial

FILIPENDULA HEXAPETALA IN CONTEMPORARY HERBALISM: Some may know of meadowsweet's role in the creation of aspirin in the mid-nineteenth century. One of the herb's chief constituents, an anti-inflammatory substance, was first isolated from the plant in the 1830s. Some sixty years later the pharmaceutical company Bayer had fabricated acetylsalicylate, a similar but artificial substance. The name aspirin comes from one of meadowsweet's older Latin names, Spiraea, and some even call the plant "herbal aspirin."[178]

Western herbalists of the second half of the twentieth century have expanded meadowsweet's healing repertoire, discoursing on its abilities for treating gout, stomachache, diarrhea, dizziness, migraine, and menopausal symptoms. In addition they value the herb as a diuretic, for reducing edema, soothing rheumatism, and addressing kidney ailments, including clearing stones. The plant has also been known to heal wounds and ulcers, to staunch hemorrhages of the respiratory system, and to stimulate the heart.[179]

Others have pointed out its strength as an antidote for counteracting poisons in addition to infections, not to mention infectious diseases such as influenza, measles, and scarlet fever. It is helpful against fever as a sudorific, and it is sometimes used as an ingredient in herbal beers.[180]

By the twenty-first century meadowsweet has become part of the herbalist's regular repertoire and continues to be described as one of the best digestive remedies available. Preparations of the herb can be applied in many conditions, including soothing the mucous membranes of the digestive tract, reducing stomach acidity, easing nausea and heartburn, reducing fevers, and soothing rheumatic pain, among its other benefits. Meadowsweet is also considered gentle enough to ease children's diarrhea.[181]

In the British Isles, while dropwort's (*Filipendula hexapetala*) roots are sometimes eaten as vegetables,[182] meadowsweet (*F. ulmaria*) is used in folk medicine for fevers, coughs, colds, sore throats, headaches, burning or itching eyes, diarrhea, generalized pain, nervousness, dropsy, kidney trouble, scrofula, and in children, jaundice.[183] It is also given to calves to relieve diarrhea.[184]

American herbalists also praise meadowsweet for its cooling and drying properties, and remind those who try the herb that its pain-relieving qualities, while similar to aspirin and without the negative side effects, take several hours to kick in. They also caution against its use in small children suffering from colds, flu, or chickenpox.[185]

In Ukraine of the mid-twentieth century, a decoction of meadowsweet flowers, bearberry leaves, corn silk, elderberry root, birch buds, horsetail, knotweed, cornflower, and several other herbs was part of a folk medicine formula used to treat diseases of the genitourinary tract along with dropsy and rheumatism.[186]

Russian herbalists associate meadowsweet with a folktale in which a knight, wracked by doubts about his ability to go into battle, is given a garland of meadowsweet flowers by a mysterious beautiful girl, and only then, consequently, is he able to defeat the invading force. Partially because of this legend, Russian folk healers recommended preparations of the herb for nervous disorders, hypertension, inflammations of the kidney and bladder, and respiratory ailments such as cough, bronchitis, bronchial asthma, tonsillitis, influenza, and the common cold. Russian healers also find the herb helpful in stomach and duodenal ulcers, dysentery, and gout. Additionally an infusion or ointment is used to relieve arthritic and skin conditions; these preparations have also been used to treat foot odor.[187]

In 2015 Serbian researchers dusted off their old herbals and set their sights once again on that oft-neglected relative of meadowsweet, dropwort (*Filipendula hexapetala*). Their study aimed to investigate the antioxidant activities of the plant, specifically its antimicrobial and antifungal abilities. It will not surprise any herbalists reading this far to learn that the researchers' very thorough and detailed study revealed what folk practitioners in Eastern Europe have known for centuries: "Aerial parts and roots of *F. hexapetala* possess remarkable antioxidant activities . . . our results imply that above ground plant parts of *F. hexapetala* could be recommended for human usage as a rich source of natural antioxidants."[188]

FILIPENDULA HEXAPETALA IN EUROPEAN HERBALISM IN THE EARLY TWENTIETH CENTURY: In the British Isles meadowsweet's aromatic, astringent, and diuretic qualities made it a valuable medicine for diarrhea; it was also nourishing as well as astringing for the bowels. Further, meadowsweet was considered of service to the stomach and was understood to be a good remedy in urinary conditions such as strangury and dropsy. And, most likely because of its gentle nature mentioned earlier, it was judged almost a specific in children's diarrhea.

Unlike other more popular applications, its support of the blood is mentioned by Maude Grieve as an alterative. Curiously she also includes its attribute as a sudorific but says that the root, decocted in white wine, was no longer considered a specific for fever. Could this have been due to the relatively recent, at the time, promotion of aspirin for treating the same condition?[189]

As noted in the Serbian study, dropwort has had a long history of use in folk medicine in many Eastern European countries: Serbia, Poland, Russia, Romania, and others. In these countries dropwort was relied on for its ability to help with rheumatism as a diuretic, as an astringent for hemorrhoids, and to treat hemorrhages, influenza, gout, inflammations, wounds, fevers, and pains in general among its other merits.[190]

In German folk medicine the roots of dropwort were used in the treatment of genitourinary and respiratory diseases.[191]

In Slovakia, however, the above-ground parts of dropwort's cousin, meadowsweet, were decocted to wash ulcers and the roots of the plant were used for urinary tract ailments.[192]

In Russian folk medicine dropwort was considered a powerful diuretic and was also known to treat rheumatism, gout, neuritis, stomach ailments, hemorrhoids, diarrhea, and hernias. Externally a decoction of the roots was applied to wounds, boils, fistulas, and ulcers.[193]

FILIPENDULA HEXAPETALA IN ASHKENAZI HERBALISM IN THE PALE IN THE EARLY TWENTIETH CENTURY:[194] Between the world wars dropwort was an herb much respected in the small Ashkenazi settlements of the Pale. The odorless knots on the rootstocks, which produce a bitter, tart taste, were gathered in May. In official state medicine dropwort had formerly been used as a strong diuretic and as a remedy for hemorrhoids, leucorrhea, and rabies.

Folk healers in the fifteen towns of Korosten, Anapol, Polona, Zhitomir, Lachovitz, Ritzev, Bazilia, Kresilev, Khmelnik, Barditchev, Ladizhin, Cherkoss, Broslev, Monasterishtche, and Savran administered a decoction of the entire plant, including the rootstock knots, or of the rootstock knots alone to those suffering from stomach and intestinal ailments, stomachache and cramps, and chronic diarrhea. To this brew they occasionally added the bark of an old oak (*Quercus robur*) and the rootstock of *Bistorta officinalis* (bistort, a plant native to Europe and commonly used to treat wounds).

A healer in the town of Litin mixed a blend of dropwort's rootstock knots and the roots of *Potentilla alba* (white cinquefoil) and *Angelica sylvestris* (wild angelica, the roots of which have been used in traditional Austrian medicine internally as tea or tincture to remedy disorders of the gastrointestinal tract, respiratory tract, and nervous system and also employed against fever, infections, and flu)[195] to create a tincture to stimulate the appetite of those unable to eat.

In Broslev an infusion or decoction of the rootstock knots or of the whole plant was a folk healer's remedy for heart diseases.

In Bohslov a traditional healer steeped the rootstock knots of dropwort in vodka together with *Falcaria vulgaris* (sickleweed) and *Valeriana* sp. (valerian) to relieve pain in the chest caused by heart diseases.

This same formulation was also known and given by folk healers in the six towns of Kresilev, Ritzev, Slavuta, Anapol, Polona, and Olt-Kosntin to members of their community who suffered from pain in "the pit of the stomach."

Dropwort was used in the treatment of kidney diseases as a diuretic in Kolenivka.

For gynecological diseases a midwife in Letichev—recall Sarah Gershenzwit Pulier, memorialized in *The Road from Letichev*—gave a dropwort preparation to new mothers for complications after childbirth, an exact replica of the remedy described almost two thousand years earlier by Dioscorides in his *materia medica*.[196]

In Bohslov a midwife made a decoction prepared from dropwort rootstock knots, the entire plant of *Falcaria vulgaris* (sickleweed or longleaf), *Valeriana* sp. (valerian) roots, and *Armoracia rusticana* (horseradish) roots, then added this strong tea to a bath for women in labor in case of complications.

A tincture of rootstock knots was given to drink in Zvenigorodka for swellings and edema due to malnutrition, and in Olt-Kosntin and Bazilia the same drink was given to remedy colds.

A rootstock tincture was given to those suffering from the pain of overexertion from having to lift and carry heavy weights in the towns of Slavuta and Olt-Kosntin.

In Bohslov a decoction or a tincture with the roots of *Falcaria vulgaris* (sickleweed), *Filipendula hexapetala* (dropwort), and *Valeriana* sp. (valerian) was prescribed by a folk healer for rheumatic pain and colds.[197]

10
FRAGARIA VESCA

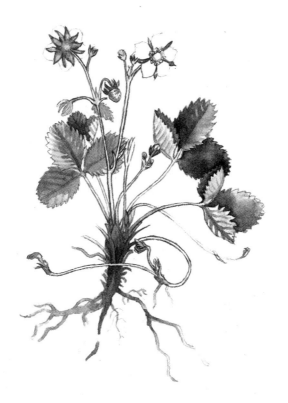

FAMILY: Rosaceae

COMMON ENGLISH NAMES: strawberry, wild strawberry, mountain strawberry, woodland strawberry, alpine strawberry, Carpathian strawberry, European strawberry

YIDDISH: פּאָזעמקע, נערד-יאַגדעס, ראַיטע יאַגדעס יאַגדעס, פּאָזיאָמכע, קלובניק, פּאָזשעמקע, פּאַטשומקע

HEBREW: תּוּת ,תּוּת ,תּוּת הַיַעַר

UKRAINIAN: Суниця, суниці лісові, суничник, позьомки, полуниці, лісна полуниця, полуничник, ягоди, червоні ягоди, ягідник, земляника

GERMAN: Erdbeere

POLISH: Poziomka pospolita

RUSSIAN: Земляника лесная, земляника обыкновенная

LITHUANIAN: Paprastoji žemuogė

DESCRIPTION AND LOCATION: Perennial found mostly in shady wild places across northern Eurasia and throughout North America. Leaves and flowers grow directly out of the rootstalk on long thin stems as do long rooting runners. Thin, light-green leaves are divided into three leaflets with roughly serrated edges and light hairs covering the underside of the leaves or their veins. As with other members of the rose family, the strawberry also produces five-petaled flowers. These small, white blooms appear from March through August and grow in clusters that rise from thin, drooping stalks above the leaves. A berry forms from the enlarged flowering end of the stalk, bearing tiny seed-like fruits on its surface.[198]

FRAGARIA VESCA **EARLY REMEDIES:**

> *The strawberry grows underneath the Nettle*
> *And wholesome berries thrive and ripen best*
> *Neighbour'd by fruit of lesser quality.*
> —William Shakespeare

Strawberries have been known since antiquity but are only mentioned in passing by classical authors such as Virgil or Pliny the Elder. In English the plant's name was originally *strewberry* because its fruit appeared to have been scattered or strewn amongst its foliage. The plant's presence in art has historically symbolized anything from sensuality and earthly desires to righteousness.[199]

Hildegard wrote that the herb on which wild strawberries (or *erpere*, as the plant was known to her) grow is more warm than cold, yet she did not favor this herb. She warned against its use as medicine because she believed it created mucus in the body and the fruit was "not good for a healthy or sick person to eat because they grow near the earth and because they also grow in putrid air."[200]

The physician Tobias ha-Kohen mentions the plant[201] as a digestive aid supporting the healthy development of the sperm and egg.[202]

In Poland the plant's healing traditions go back centuries, if not millennia. Wild strawberries are believed to have grown in the region since Neolithic times and served as food for early Slavs. By the sixteenth century Polish physicians were noting preparations of strawberry could treat lung and pancreas inflammations, reduce high fevers, and rid the mouth of bad tastes. The plant was also sought to extract the poison from a spider bite, quell rashes, soothe sore eyes, ease colds, reduce kidney and gallbladder stones, heal burns, and treat jaundice and scurvy. In addition the root never failed to staunch a nosebleed when placed in an affected nostril. Roma living in Poland were known to use wild strawberries as a general appetite stimulant and gave them to anemic children. The plant also served culinary needs as an addition to broths or syrups.[203]

FRAGARIA VESCA **CONTEMPORARY ACTIONS:** astringent, diuretic, tonic

FRAGARIA VESCA **CONTEMPORARY MEDICINAL PARTS:** whole plant

FRAGARIA VESCA **IN CONTEMPORARY HERBALISM:** American herbalists in the 1970s were aware that a tea made from the strawberry's leaves and roots was beneficial to those experiencing diarrhea, dysentery, hematuria, urinary tract gravel, and other discomforts of the urinary system. For skin conditions such as acne or eczema, drinking the tea while simultaneously bathing affected areas with it topically could provide some relief. To cool a feverish condition, the fresh juice from the fruit has been found helpful. A tea made from the leaf was also said to be a tonic in convalescence and safe for children.[204]

The Indigenous peoples of North America have found all parts of the plant to remedy diarrhea and dysentery. For stomach disorders a root tea was prepared. Sores were treated with a poultice of the leaves.[205]

Girls in early twentieth-century Cornwall applied the leaves of this plant to improve their complexions; the source of such a remedy may possibly have been a technique gleaned from a folk song that originated in that region. In Ireland some believe that strawberry leaf tea could quell "excessive ardor."[206]

In Poland the leaves of wild strawberry are mixed with those of raspberry; the blend is considered one of the best substitutes for regular tea.[207] In Russia the fruit is currently recommended to treat sclerosis, high blood pressure (hypertension), constipation, intestinal ailments, and diarrhea.[208]

In contemporary Lithuanian official medicine, strawberries have been considered a valuable healing plant. As a part of a healthy diet, strawberries are a source of vitamin C, and a leaf infusion can treat cardiovascular disease and support digestion and liver and kidney function by eliminating toxins and reducing cholesterol. For oral health a rinse with the fresh juice is recommended to reduce inflammation of the mucous membranes or to eliminate any harmful microbes that cause bad breath. Leaf and berry infusions are drunk to relieve gout. Berries, high in iron, are taken to remedy anemia. Infusions of the dried fruit relieve fever and promote sweating, and can help to break up kidney and gallbladder stones, or treat scurvy and gout. The fruits are part of a helpful regimen to treat intestinal tract inflammations, hemorrhoids, tuberculosis, and diabetes. Dental tartar can be reduced by chewing strawberries as well.

Folk medicine practitioners in Lithuania also work with this plant for healing heart disease, hypertension, atherosclerosis, stones, and colds, among other health concerns. As a cosmetic ingredient, a paste of the leaves and fresh berries is compounded into facial exfoliating masks by mixing with egg whites. Fresh berry juice is also used to fade freckles, blemishes, and acne. A leaf decoction is used to treat rashes, acne, and scrofula.[209]

Those considering ingesting the strawberry are warned by all sources that some people may have an allergic reaction to the plant.

FRAGARIA VESCA IN EUROPEAN HERBALISM IN THE EARLY TWENTIETH CENTURY: The British herbalist Maude Grieve, writing in the first decades of the twentieth century, mentions that because the wild strawberry is much smaller and more dainty than its cultivated cousin, it yields a more delicate and exquisite flavor. Regardless of these subtle qualities, in the British Isles the plant served as laxative, diuretic, and astringent. In early English pharmacopoeias, while the fruit and leaves were included, it was the latter that were called upon most.

For fevers the fruit was taken to cool the condition. The root was used to astringe diarrhea as was the tea, which was taken to check dysentery.

For oral health it was known that the plant's fresh fruit whitened the teeth if the juice was held in the mouth for several minutes then rinsed with warm water. To clear the skin and soothe a mild sunburn, a freshly cut fruit was rubbed over the face immediately after washing. For a more intense sunburn the juice was worked into the skin, left on for thirty minutes, then washed off with warm water to which were added a few drops of tincture of benzoin (a pungent ethanol solution of benzoin resin from the bark of several species of trees in the genus *Styrax*).[210]

Bavarians at the turn of the twentieth century found strawberries helpful to warm frozen feet by putting on, barefoot, a pair of boots filled with the berries for a few hours to thaw the extremities. The same condition was also treated with dried strawberries. This unique remedy may have its explanation in the fact that the fruit ripens just when the frosts are thawing and therefore can lessen the effects one may experience during this transitional season.[211]

Slovaks were known to crush the early fruits with their fingers and smear the juice on freckles, hoping to fade them. To treat haemoptysis, strawberry roots were cut into sticks to make a tea. Young leaves were also taken as tea for the same condition. In Russia at the end of the nineteenth century, to expel intestinal worms patients were advised to eat herring daily with onions, garlic, and lots of strawberries.[212]

Long-standing cases of eczema, especially those that could not be cured by various expensive means, were successfully treated by wild strawberries. This method involved rubbing a thick layer of the fresh fruit on a clean linen cloth. Repeated daily application of such a poultice placed on affected areas cleared them of scabs, eliminated fluid congestion, removed any foul odor, and prepared the area for applying cooling lotions.

In addition Russian folk healers made infusions from dried leaves and the rhizome for treating blemishes, scrofula, rickets, gout, gastritis, menorrhagia, jaundice, hemorrhoids, anemia, and liver, spleen, and intestinal diseases.[213]

A well-known Soviet authority who spent many years studying the health benefits of strawberries praised the plant, stating that it should be of interest to researchers and practitioners with a special focus on the plant's benefit to the urinary system, in addition to its helpfulness against liver disease, gallstones, stomach catarrhs, and diseases of the spleen. The same herbalist noted that strawberry cures were popular among the people, specifically those who did not have the means to take cures at spas and resorts. One such folk remedy called for infusing fifty grams of strawberries per liter of water to cleanse the blood and treat rashes, pimples, herpes, rickets, gout, gastritis, diseases of the liver and spleen, catarrh of the colon, hemorrhoids, and jaundice.[214]

And as a widely quoted Russian proverb puts it, "In the house where strawberries and blueberries are eaten, the doctor has nothing to do."

FRAGARIA VESCA **IN ASHKENAZI HERBALISM IN THE PALE IN THE EARLY TWENTIETH CENTURY:**[215] In the Pale at the turn of the twentieth century, wild strawberries were abundant, growing in forests and meadows and common in places where many Ashkenazi communities flourished. In folk medicine the berries, rootstock, and leaves were widely employed. Many of the following remedies are very similar to those used in Lithuania and other parts of the Pale of Settlement.

A decoction of the above-ground portion of the plant with the berries was drunk as a remedy for kidney disease in Romen. By adding the rootstock to this tea, it was used to quell catarrh of the stomach and intestines in both Yelisavetgrod and Ladizhin.

An infusion of the dried leaves, at times with berries mixed in, was drunk like a tea for pain in the chest or cough in several towns and villages including Barditchev, Olt-Kosntin, Polona, Lachovitz, Ritzev, Monasterishtche, Broslev, Zhitomir, and Cherkoss. In Kiev this mixture was taken to strengthen the heart.

Folk healers in Yelisavetgrod combined the rootstocks, leaves, and berries as a decoction for gallstones. In the same town the berries were a remedy for bladder stones and, in a formula identical to that of the Roma of Poland, the fruits were known as a remedy to stimulate the metabolism in those with anemia.

For colds and high fevers, traditional healers in Kiev, Zhitomir, Kharkov, Olt-Kosntin, Ritzev, Polona, and Lachovitz gave a decoction or strong infusion of the whole plant, including the roots, to drink.

A warm decoction was used for gargling in case of diptheria in Zhitomir.

The berries were recommended as a remedy for nervous disorders in Polona. In Yelisavetgrod, Polona, and Korosten the berries and rootstocks were a remedy for insomnia, and combined with the leaves they were used for neurasthenia in those towns as well.

A decoction of flowers, berries, and roots was used to wash the head and invigorate the scalp in Kiev.

In Polona a leaf and root infusion was given to children suffering from whooping cough and colds.

11

HYPERICUM PERFORATUM

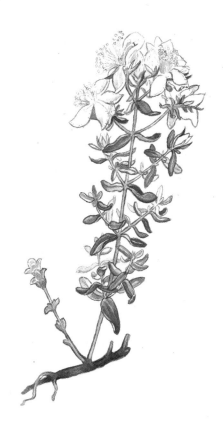

FAMILY: Hypericaceae

COMMON ENGLISH NAMES: Common St. John's wort

YIDDISH: שדים-שוצ ,יאהאנעס קרייטער

HEBREW: פרעא ,פרע

UKRAINIAN: Заяча крівця звичайна, заяча кровця, Божа крівця, крівця, крівавник, кровавник, кровавець, крівавець, кроволин, кровопій, світоянське зілля, свістоянське зілля, свентоянське зілля, жовте свентоянське зілля, звіробой, звіробой тонколистий, звіробій, зверобой, громобой, жовте зілля, пожарниця, покровка

GERMAN: Johanniskraut

POLISH: Dziurawiec zwyczajny, dzwonki Panny Marii, ziele Świętego Jana, krewka Matki Boskiej, dziurawiec pospolity, ruta polna, krzyżowe ziele, arlika, przestrzelon

RUSSIAN: Зверобой обыкновенный

LITHUANIAN: Paprastoji Jonažolė

DESCRIPTION AND LOCATION: Shrub-like perennial found in undeveloped gravelly areas, woods, fields, meadows, and along roads throughout Eurasia and coastal North America. From the base of woody roots grow round, erect, branching stems that send out runners. Leaves grow opposite each other along slender upright branches and are pale green, oblong, and dotted with small dark oil glands that are visible by holding the leaf to light. Five-petaled warm yellow flowers, also speckled with black dots and lines, contain an oil that produces a red liquid when crushed. The plant blooms from June to September, eventually yielding small, round, black seeds within capsules that have a resinous smell and a bitter, astringent, and balsamic taste. The plant as a whole smells of turpentine.[216]

***HYPERICUM PERFORATUM* EARLY REMEDIES:** Many ancient superstitions are associated with St. John's wort. Its name, *Hypericum*, originates with the Greeks and translates as "over an apparition," which is an allusion to the belief that the plant was so objectionable to evil spirits that even a whiff of it could cause them to flee.[217] A Yiddish name for this plant, *shedim shuts*, literally "demon protection," succinctly reiterates this sentiment.

St. John's wort has been used in folk medicine to treat external wounds for thousands of years. The first documentation of its healing properties can be found in the works of Hippocrates and Theophrastus.[218]

In the first century Dioscorides was pragmatic in his description of St. John's wort and singled the herb out for its "hip ailment" affinities, its ability to draw out bilious matter and excrement, and its healing strength when plastered on burns.[219] Subsequently Galen added a note about its astringency and stimulating properties for urination.[220] But later, Hildegard, who knew the plant as "*harte-nauwe*," singled out its cold character and deemed the plant worthy only as animal fodder because it was so uncultivated and neglected as an herb.[221]

Writing in the Islamic world, Maimonides recorded the plant's names, which differed markedly from the Greek. In Arabic and Spanish, St. John's wort was associated with meanings like "forgetful," "which appeases grief," "calming," and "heart herb."[222]

The English botanist John Gerard contributed his thoughts on the plant's protective qualities, explaining that "if placed in a room it will guard the inmate from all evil influences."[223] Paracelsus in his time also mentioned the herb's protective properties, but with respect to the preservation of cheese. He noted that if the herb were placed against the food, the wort could protect it against worms, and if touched by the plant, the infestors would die and drop out of their host. He also commented on the fact that the plant's specific name, *perforatum*, similar to other plants with distinguishing physical characteristics, was so called because of holes lining the margins of its leaves.[224]

The physician Tobias ha-Kohen also found *Hypericum* of value, mentioning the plant's effect on the urinary system and possibly citing its ability to treat stones. More than once he referred to the herb's effectiveness in addressing digestive troubles.[225]

During the Middle Ages and afterward, Poles believed that the plant cured ninety-nine illnesses in addition to its powers against magic and evil forces. If hung in a window, it was thought to protect the home against lightning. Medicinally, Polish folk healers found it to be a diuretic and wound healing herb when its fresh flowers were infused in spirytus and then applied to lacerations, burns, and ulcers.[226]

HYPERICUM PERFORATUM **CONTEMPORARY ACTIONS:** antiseptic, astringent, vulnerary, anti-anxiety, antidepressant, anti-inflammatory, antiviral, digestive tonic, nervine

HYPERICUM PERFORATUM **CONTEMPORARY MEDICINAL PARTS:** aerial, or above-ground, parts

HYPERICUM PERFORATUM **IN CONTEMPORARY HERBALISM:** St. John's wort is a revered folk medicine wherever it grows and has been in continual use since at least the time of the ancients. A cross-cultural survey of the plant's medicinal application in the late twentieth century records its use in Azerbaijan for intestinal disorders, as an analgesic for abdominal pain, and as a tonic and sedative for nervous disorders; in North America Native people heal snake bites with the plant; traditional healers in France use the plant to treat burns; in Bulgaria it has long been sought for gastric acidity reduction, gout, sciatica, rheumatism, hemorrhoids, children's bed-wetting, diarrhea, and nervous disorders; in the British Isles the plant has topical applications for skin lesions and internal applications for intestinal worms; folk healers in Lithuania and Ukraine have found a remedy in the plant for cancer of the liver, stomach, ovaries, and goiter; in Moldova chronic colitis, gingivitis, and stomatitis are treated by traditional practitioners with St. John's wort; and in Uzbekistan an oil preparation helps with skin diseases.[227] In contemporary officially recognized medicine and as an ingredient in commercial healing products, *Hypericum perforatum* is also valued by the French, Czechs, Romanians, Poles, and Germans.[228]

"It is as impossible to make bread without flour as it is to heal people without St. John's wort." This Russian proverb attests to the plant's importance in that country's healing history.[229] In traditional medicine in Russia, an incredible assortment of preparations with this herb have treated asthma, colds, gastric and duodenal ulcers, and scurvy.[230] It has been employed to promote the flow and filtration of urine, help with the flow of bile from the gallbladder, relieve a variety of pulmonary complaints, treat gout and rheumatism, and ease nervous tension, headaches, insomnia, chest congestion, tuberculosis, and hemorrhoids. A topical oil infusion remedies burns, sores, and wounds, while a tincture can be gargled to treat sores in the mouth.

With regard to St. John's wort, contemporary Lithuanian folk medicine application is similar to that of Russia, with several additions including as a healing agent for malignant tumors and to reduce inflammation, relieve pain, stop spasms, staunch bleeding, and stimulate circulation.[231]

Because research in the last decades of the twentieth century touted St. John's wort as being effective for mild depression, commercial preparations of the herb have become popular in the United States. American herbalists, however, know this herb as having many more virtues with regard to human health. Among these, the herb is looked to for help with insomnia, anxiety, nerve damage, and wound repair. Its antiviral properties can assist with infections such as shingles, herpes, mononucleosis, and influenza.[232] Famed herbalist Rosemary Gladstar writes of St. John's wort's uplifting properties, and she reminds us that the actions of this herb are not fully understood in the scientific community, and that it is in the whole plant, not its isolated constituent parts, where St. John's wort's healing powers lie.[233]

All herbalists note that while *Hypericum* has a multitude of healing powers, it must be applied with care. It should not be taken with SSRI antidepressants, and because it is phototoxic, it will cause skin sensitivity in those taking it if they are exposed to sunlight.

HYPERICUM PERFORATUM IN EUROPEAN HERBALISM OF THE EARLY TWENTIETH CENTURY: Belief in *Hypericum*'s powers was great and widespread in early twentieth-century Europe. Its names were numerous; some English translations of the various foreign titles include hard hay, spotted hard hay, devil's flight, elf blood, Christ's cruciferous blood, Our Lord's blood herb, Our Lord's wounds, St. John's blood, and witch's herb.

In the Havel region of eastern Germany, a little verse summoning the power of Hartenaus—the same name for the herb that Hildegard had used a thousand years before—was sung during thunderstorms to keep danger away. People there protected their cattle against bewitching by burying the plant under the barn door threshold.

In Silesia the plant was an indicator of love. The color produced when the plant was crushed in one's hand determined whether affections would be returned. The ritual was accompanied by a short rhyme:

You are good to me
Give me blood
I'm sorry
Give me mud

In other parts of Germany, wreaths made with the herb were thrown on the roofs of houses to protect them from fire.

Medicinally St. John's wort was taken in the Tyrolean region to relieve fatigue. In Bavaria, soaked in oil, it was called *Johannesblut*, "John's blood," and was applied to heal wounds and rashes.

In Prussia a tea made from the herb was taken to treat colds; in addition the family and livestock were protected from harm by placing the plant around living quarters—especially if collected on the saint's day, which falls around the summer solstice.

The Slovaks believed that when the plant was picked on St. John's Day it had special powers, and it was mostly used for smoking.

The Slovenes prepared the flowers by placing them in a bottle they then covered with a fine oil. After allowing this mixture to soak in the sun for thirty days, they pressed it out through a cloth, mixed the resulting infused oil with a little camphor, rosemary oil, and juniper berry oil, then placed it back in the sun for another three days. When this process was finished, the resulting ointment was a ready remedy.[234]

In Poland up until the twentieth century, *Hypericum*, believed to protect a new mother and baby against evil spirits, was put around the house and placed around the neck of the infant until their first bath.[235]

In the Soviet Union St. John's wort was "the most important medicinal plant we knew" and was popularly called "grass that cures ninety-nine diseases," the same moniker as that of medieval Poles.

Hypericum perforatum had long been used in Russia in both folk and official medicine, both alone and in conjunction with other herbs; many preparations were relied on for treating liver disease, disorders of the stomach, intestines, bladder, and kidney, a number of gynecological disorders, lung diseases, inflammatory processes, abscesses, ulcers, boils, skin rashes, rheumatism, physical strain, gangrenous sores, and even bed-wetting and halitosis.[236]

Official Soviet pharmacology produced ointments and aerosols derived from St. John's wort to treat wounds, burns, abscesses, soft tissue inflammations, boils, mastitis, injuries to the outer eye, and diseases of the sinuses, throat, and upper airways. It was also used internally to treat irritation of the gastrointestinal tract and as a mouth rinse against stomatitis and gingivitis.[237] St. John's wort has been called the most important folk medicinal plant in the region, and a famous Ukrainian herbalist has said of it:

> *Regarding its therapeutic "strength," I personally compare St. John's wort with strawberries, with the only difference that the strawberry season lasts three to four weeks (berry season) and, when dried, strawberries mostly lose their active properties, while St. John's wort is always fresh and effective when sun-dried. I believe that in all our flora there is, in this sense, no plant like St. John's wort. The people call it "the herb of ninety-nine diseases."*[238]

HYPERICUM PERFORATUM IN ASHKENAZI HERBALISM IN THE PALE IN THE EARLY TWENTIETH CENTURY:[239] As in other parts of the Soviet Union, between the world wars traditional healers in the Pale relied on *Hypericum perforatum* as a remedy for many of the ailments their communities suffered. Out of almost one hundred towns and villages examined between the wars, the vast majority reported medicinal knowledge of St. John's wort, attesting to the herb's important role in the Eastern European folk healer's repertoire. The herb was commonly found in meadows, on hills, and among the shrubs of Ukraine.

In Letichev, Ashkenazi traditional healers treated skin disorders with the herb.[240]

Folk healers relied on preparations of St. John's wort to treat various intestinal ailments and kidney troubles in almost twenty settlements. These included Anapol, Slavuta, Polona, Lachovitz, Zaslov, Ritzev, Kresilev, Monasterishtche, Broslev, Balte, Birzula, Cherkoss, Zvenigorodka, and Konotop. Those same folk healers, plus several others in the towns of Letichev, Litin, and Konotop, most likely local feldshers, treated cases of diarrhea and bloody diarrhea using preparations of St. John's wort.

In Kolenivka a folk healer sought the plant to treat dysentery.

A seed tincture of the herb was prepared by a healer to cure diarrhea in Ulanov.

The plant tops with the flowers were used for respiratory ailments such as cough and shortness of breath, pneumonia, and lung diseases in Priluki and Ulanov.

In Zhitomir a folk healer treated tuberculosis with the plant.

For kidney, blood, and metabolic diseases, healers in Shvartz-Timeh, Savran, and Birzula turned to this herb.

For headaches caused by anemia or dizziness, a decoction of the herb either washed the hair of both the young and old afflicted with this ailment or was given as a drink by healers in Korosten, Korsn, Bohslov, Broslev, and Monasterishtche. Sometimes the folk healer in Lachovitz added *Achillea millefolium*, or yarrow, to the formula.

If a person or cow was bitten by a mad dog in Bazilia, a decoction of St. John's wort was given to help cure the infection.

In Priluki, Ritzev, Polona, and Khmelnik an ointment preparation was applied for head colds.

Fresh or festering sores in Khmelnik were treated with an ointment that combined fresh or dried flowers with butter and was applied locally.

A plant tincture was used for washing wounds in Makhnivke.

The most interesting applications of St. John's wort in the Pale are the remedies for nervous system conditions. These treatments seem to anticipate contemporary research done in the last part of the twentieth century that highlights the plant's ability to calm anxiety and depression.

For example, in Broslev a decoction of the plant was given by folk healers there as a remedy for nervous diseases, including as a massage "in case of paralysis." The word *paralysis* in association with fear was also used in the story "The Healer from Bilgoray," where it was modified by the Yiddish word *gekhapt*, or "seized."[241] This modifying of the word *paralysis* can most definitely be linked to the idea of a possession, possibly by an imagined demon—in fact, the Yiddish name for the plant, *shedim shuts*, translates to "demon protection." In the Biłgoraj story, the patient was treated by an opshprekherin who performed a ritual wax ceremony and may have also used herbs as part of her cure. Because the documentation in both the Biłgoraj story and the event recorded in Broslev are so scant, it is difficult to know the exact elements of each case. But it is extremely possible that the healer who was interviewed in Broslev was an opshprekherin and that the treatment recounted in Biłgoraj included a preparation employing St. John's wort. It is also very likely that these two Ashkenazi folk healers were attempting to cure a paralyzing fear brought on by the belief in demons or even the evil eye, both of which were common notions in the Pale at the turn of the twentieth century.

A further sign that this plant was well-known and employed by opshprekherins comes from the author of the Soviet-era ethnobotanical survey herself, Natalia Ossadcha-Janata. In an unusual aside she briefly describes how her father had suffered for years with chronic indigestion. While it's speculative to conclude his predicament was caused by stress or anxiety, the fact remains that, after trying in vain "every possible medicine," at the advice of a "village quack" her father began taking a preparation of St. John's wort, and his chronic indigestion was cured.[242] The term "quack" was often applied to a healer who did not have academic training and whose practice included both herbs and magic.

In the Pale *Hypericum* was also important to gynecological health. An infusion of the whole plant was given to women in labor by midwives in Anapol and Ritzev.

In Barditchev and Cherkoss women suffering from (unspecified) gynecological diseases were helped by this herb.

And in Bohslov the same infusion was given to induce menstruation and to stop hemorrhaging in both men and women.

For children who suffered from diarrhea, a midwife gave an herb infusion, as either a bath or a drink; in Olt-Kosntin and in Bazilia the midwife gave the same remedy to children with incontinence or bed-wetting, perhaps to treat symptoms of fear.

Many people in the Pale did backbreaking work, including lifting or hauling heavy objects, which caused overstrain and pain. For this condition a tincture was prepared using *Hypericum perforatum, Quercus robur* bark (English oak), *Prunus cerasus* bark (tart cherry), *Rheum* roots (rhubarb), *Achillea millefolium* herb (yarrow), and *Ruta graveolens* (rue) and given as a remedy in Zvenigorodka, Slavuta, Ritzev, Olt-Kosntin, Kresilev, Monasterishtche, and Broslev.

In folk veterinary medicine, a plant decoction was fed to cattle suffering from bloody urine and stomachache in Balte, Zvenigorodka, and Chopovitch.

12
LAVATERA THURINGIACA

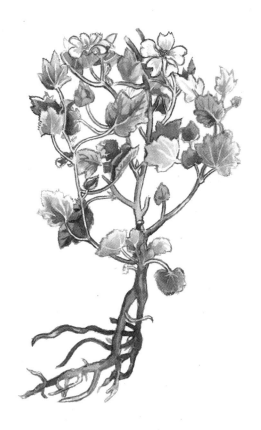

FAMILY: Malvaceae

COMMON ENGLISH NAMES: garden tree-mallow

YIDDISH: לאַוואַטערע מאַלווע,

HEBREW: אזניות

UKRAINIAN: Собача рожа, польова рожа, рожа, шелудова рожа, рожа дика, алтейний корінь

GERMAN: Thüringer Strauchpappel, Buschmalve

POLISH: Ślazówka turyngska, ślaz lekarski

RUSSIAN: Хатьма тюрингенская, собачья рожа

LITHUANIAN: Šlaitinė rožūnė

NOTE: Because Russian sources consider *Lavatera thuringiaca* as having identical medicinal properties to its mallow cousin *Althaea officinalis*, this plant profile will identify which mallow is being described and also occasionally refer to the plants interchangeably. Other herbalists corroborate the plants' identical medicinal actions, including Maurice Mességué: "all [mallows] have the same [medicinal] virtues." With this in mind, for the purposes of this plant profile, the use of garden tree-mallow in the Pale has been interchangeably noted with that of *Althaea officinalis*.[243]

DESCRIPTION AND LOCATION: *Lavatera thuringiaca*, the garden tree-mallow, is a species of Lavatera native to Eastern Europe and southwestern Asia, from southern Germany south to Italy, and east to southern Russia, Kazakhstan, and Turkey. It is an herbaceous perennial that can attain heights of close to six feet. Palm-shaped leaves with three or five lobes grow to three and a half inches in length and breadth and are covered in downy grayish hairs. The five-petaled flowers are purplish pink, one to two inches in diameter, and bloom throughout the summer months.[244]

***LAVATERA THURINGIACA* AND *ALTHAEA OFFICINALIS* EARLY REMEDIES:** Decades ago biblical scholars translated a passage in the book of Job as describing mallows as part of a meal that was eaten by the ancients in times of deprivation. But the Hebrew word invoked in the passage, *malluach*, has since been interpreted as referring to a salty plant—probably not mallows as we know them today.

It's more than a little thrilling to find that this modest herb has been honored consistently for millennia for its same healing qualities. In the early years of the first century, Dioscorides described *althaia*—which translates in English as "to heal"—as having leaves like the cyclamen, rounded but downy, flowers that are rose-like, and a root that is sticky and white inside. Mostly, though, he wrote of its ability to cure many diseases in a variety of preparations. Among the concerns the plant treated when boiled in a hydromel (a drink similar to mead, made with honey and water) or wine, or chopped and applied by itself were physical injuries, tumors, scrofula, abscesses, inflamed breasts, anal inflammations, and bruises. *Althaia* also was known to disperse "inflations" and tension in tendons by its ability to bring to a head an infection, breaking it loose and cicatrizing it (or healing it by scar formation).

Softened with pork or goose fat and turpentine, the *althaia* mixture was placed in a pessary by the ancient Greeks to soothe "uterine inflammations and closings." As a decoction it was known to accomplish the same tasks and also remove the "discharges of childbirth."

Drunk with wine, a decoction of its root benefitted those with difficulty urinating, kidney stones, hip ailments, dysentery, "quivering," and ruptures. When boiled with vinegar and used as a rinse, it soothed toothaches. Even the seeds, fresh or dry, were ground in vinegar and then smeared on "dull-white leprosies." Infections from animal attacks were protected against with an ointment of the seeds steeped in vinegar and oil. This same concoction was recommended for dysentery, the coughing up of blood, and diarrhea. A decoction of the seeds was drunk for those suffering from bee stings, and the same brew was combined with sour wine and then drunk for "the strokes of all small animals." Even the leaves were plastered on bites and burns with a little olive oil.

Almost as an afterthought Dioscorides noted that the root, when ground up in water and placed in the sun, was observed to thicken the liquid. Little did Dioscorides know this would be *althaia*'s most cherished attribute, the one contemporary herbalists would turn to again and again for so many of the remedies we know today.[245]

A century later Galen wrote about the herb, this time stressing the power of the root, in addition to the whole plant, to mildly yet effectively loosen and soften stiffness and localized hardening of the body's soft tissues.[246]

The abbess Hildegard wrote of "*ybischa*," as she knew the plant in midtwelfth-century Germany, as hot and dry. She prescribed pounding the herb in vinegar and drinking it, followed by fasting in the morning and night, for those with fevers of any kind. For someone with headaches, she recommended crushing together *ybischa* plus a little less sage mixed with olive oil. This ointment was to be warmed in the hands near a fire then tied into place on the forehead, for both pain relief and improved sleep.[247]

Around the same time Hildegard was setting down her observations, the plant was included in most European pharmacopoeias. Maimonides, in his glossary of *materia medica*, identified the herb in Arabic as *hitmi* (the equivalent to the Greek *althaia*) where, in the Maghrib, or northwestern Africa, it was known as the "rose of prostitutes." In the Arab lands the flowers were gathered a little before their opening, dried, and sold in the drug bazaars under the name *hatmi*. Also in the Near East by that time, as in Europe, the herb served as a pectoral and bechic, or cough reliever.[248]

By the early 1700s, when the physician Tobias ha-Kohen published his work, he included many references to the humble mallow. In his Hebrew text, the herb can be found transliterated as *"altia,"* and its healing powers include the treatment of asthma and dryness along with the herbs *Marrubium vulgare* (white horehound), *Tussilago farfara* (coltsfoot), and licorice; its root he mixed with other plants as a bandage to soften inflammations, and he also recommended the plant for urinary concerns, and for pain and swelling. In a further harkening back to the ancients, ha-Kohen included *altia* as a softening medicine to be combined with other herbs as a gynecological treatment for easing the birthing process.[249]

Samuel-Auguste Tissot's best-selling medical reference, *Advice to the People*, published in 1761 (and translated into Yiddish "Taytsch" by Moses Marcuse in 1790), mentioned marshmallow in four formulations. In the original recommendations an ointment of marshmallow was prescribed for rheumatism's stiffness in the joints, but only after a steam of the affected area was dried off with hot linen. For an "inflammatory cholic" a glyster (also known as *clyster*: cleansing medicines injected into the rectum through clyster pipes or syringes) containing a decoction of mallows was to be given every two hours.

In addressing women wishing to ease delivery during a difficult childbirth, Tissot, in sync with ha-Kohen, adhered to the prescriptions of the ancients, openly chastising any midwife who may have offered her patient some relief with a calming herbal tincture of the mallow. Instead, he urged that every fourth hour a glyster consisting of a decoction of the herb with a little bit of oil be inserted into the laboring woman to ease the birth process. Whether this was for the attending physician's benefit or that of the patient, Tissot did not specify.

For teething children in pain, Tissot also recommended this same decoction and administration.

He also wrote that a decoction of the herb be taken when an object was blocking the throat, to soften and smooth the irritated parts and loosen the obstructing body.[250]

Tissot also looked to mallow for burns, wounds, contusions or bruises, sprains, ulcers, frostbitten limbs, chilblains, ruptures and boils, felons, thorns or splinters, warts, and corns. For poisons inflaming the digestive tract, a healing demulcent was advised, and marshmallow was thought the most suitable.[251]

ALTHAEA OFFICINALIS **CONTEMPORARY ACTIONS:** anodyne, demulcent, emollient, expectorant, diuretic, galactagogue, nutritive, vulnerary

ALTHAEA OFFINALIS **CONTEMPORARY MEDICINAL PARTS:** root, leaf

ALTHAEA OFFICINALIS **IN CONTEMPORARY HERBALISM:** Contemporary herbalists the world over find the mallows' powers excel in their moisturizing properties, both as an emollient (external) and a demulcent (internal). In the United States the famed "godmother of herbalism," Rosemary Gladstar, has suggested serving marshmallow tea for sore throats, diarrhea, constipation, or bronchial inflammation. Externally she describes a paste made with the powdered root for relieving irritated skin; or added to a bath with oatmeal, it can provide a soothing wash.[252]

In the British Isles, records from Norfolk show the fruits of a mallow, possibly *Malva sylvestris*, for their laxative properties are given to children to chew, while in three other English regions mallow has long had a good reputation as a general cleanser of the system. It is proposed that these uses may be traced back as early as pre-Roman folk medicine.

Generally, however, in the British Isles *Malvaceae* have been sought for two ailments, one external and the other internal. The more common of the two is as a soothing poultice for skin irritations or inflammations of any kind, as well as to soften and disperse swellings. In some regions, not only the leaves but sometimes the roots or flowers are pounded and mixed with lard or goose grease to make a "marshmallow salve." The herb's second popular application has been to treat coughs, colds, sore throats, asthma, and chest troubles. For these complaints the plant is chewed, sucked, infused, drunk, or gargled with. A third less-reported application has been for easing rheumatic complaints; for these a poultice is applied. A few other remedies employing mallows have been recorded, such as for sore or strained eyes, varicosities, toothache and teething, kidney and urinary troubles, dysentery, corns, gripes in children, and gonorrhea. It is noted that at times in its folk medicine, mallow may have served as an alternative to comfrey when the latter was not available.[253]

Under the entry for marshmallow root (*Althaea officinalis*) in the index of the British text *Principles and Practices of Phytotherapy*, the authors list fourteen separate entries for this herb: acute bronchitis, antitussive properties, chronic bronchitis/emphysema, chronic tonsillitis, dyspepsia, food intolerance/allergy, gastroenteritis, gastroesophageal reflux, hyperlipidaemia, mucilages, poultices, respiratory demulcent properties, sore throat, and urinary tract infection.[254]

Livestock in Poland find relief from wounds when their caregivers wash them with a light decoction of marshmallow and chamomile.[255]

In contemporary Russia the perennial plant both grows in the wild and is cultivated by herbalists throughout the country. Folk healers have traditionally used all of the plant's parts, but official state medicine has focused exclusively on its root, where the mucilage and essential oils are concentrated. Its healing properties soothe mucosa, protecting the body's tissues from irritation. Russian researchers have detected a relationship between the stomach's hydrochloric acid and the physical properties of mallow, noting that if mallow is taken when stomach acid is increased, the plant's mucilage thickens, better protecting the mucus layers in the stomach. Those with gastritis, stomach ulcers, and other irritations in the digestive tract are treated with this herb. Other preparations are applied for quinsy (abscesses of the tonsillar area), jaundice, kidney stones, difficult urination, inflamed eyelids, inflammations of the upper respiratory system, and sore throat. The plant is also used in conjunction with other medications in Russia for the treatment of pneumonia. Herbalists recommend harvesting the leaves and flowers in summer, although the roots can be collected in either spring or fall and should be peeled before using.[256]

A well-known contemporary German herbalist advises a "Cough Tea No. 1" formula that includes mallows for the treatment of bronchitis, and reminds readers that the anti-inflammatory herb specifically inhibits bacterial growth while coating and protecting inflamed mucous membranes.[257]

***LAVATERA THURINGIACA* AND *ALTHAEA OFFICINALIS* IN EUROPEAN HERBALISM IN THE EARLY TWENTIETH CENTURY:** In Russian folk medicine, preparations from *Lavatera thuringiaca* were used for diseases of the airways, coughs, colds, and various ailments of the digestive tract; its action was considered very close to marshmallow.[258]

Elsewhere in Europe in the early twentieth century, preparations of marshmallow, with its soothing qualities, were still very much in use by country people especially for relief of inflammation, both externally and internally. The plant was also used in lozenge formulas. French druggists and English sweetmeat-makers at the turn of the previous century prepared a paste from the roots of the herb, *pâté de guimauve,* in contrast to the fluffy white sugar blobs we roast over campfires today. Its emollient properties were soothing to a sore chest and valued for the relief of coughs and hoarseness.

In France the young tops and leaves of the marshmallow were part of a spring salad known to stimulate the kidneys. For the same healing purpose a syrup was prepared from the roots.[259]

Poles drank a decoction of the root for a cough, cold, or difficult breathing. The plant's fresh leaves were applied to sores and boils, and for swollen glands in the neck, the leaves were steeped and placed on the affected area.[260]

For a hernia, the herb was finely minced with both anise and mint then combined with rye flour and fat. This paste was then applied to a cloth that was placed on the hernia. The herb's flowers along with linden were infused in honey to treat colds.[261]

In Tyrolia the root and leaves of *Eibisch*—a word similar to the *ybischa* known by Hildegard von Bingen—were known as a healing medicine.

The Czechs created a mixture of linden flowers, nettles, nettle roots, licorice, and marshmallow for a cough medicine. In Moravia for the same complaint, a mixture of sugar, fennel or licorice, marshmallow root, lungwort (*Pulmonaria officinalis*), sage (*Salvia officinalis*), mullein (*Verbascum phlomoides*), and heath speedwell (*Veronica officinalis*) was decocted in milk, water, or wine. If accompanying chest pain was very severe, butter was added as well.

In Styria in the Austrian Alps, not far from Slovenia, catarrhs of the airways were treated with sweat cures, but "moisturizing, expectorant" teas also played a role. One combination included elderberry (*Sambucus nigra*), mullein (*Verbascum thapsus*), linden blossom (*Tilia europaea*), and marshmallow root, among other demulcent herbs.

LAVATERA THURINGIACA **IN ASHKENAZI HERBALISM IN THE PALE IN THE EARLY TWENTIETH CENTURY:**[262] *Lavatera thuringiaca*, or garden tree-mallow, was common in meadows and as a weed on farms everywhere in the Pale.

For colds, chest pain, coughs, sore throat, and tuberculosis, a decoction of the roots or the leaves and flowers was administered as a drink by folk healers in Kresilev, Broslev, Birzula, Zvenigorodka, Bohslov, Barditchev, and Letichev.

Also in Letichev, as in other parts of the Podolia region, mallow was a remedy for sore throats, toothaches, upset stomachs, and burns.[263]

In Cherkoss a root decoction was taken as a gargle against catarrh.

A traditional healer in Balte applied the boiled, crushed root to the chest (poultice) for those suffering pain in the throat due to diphtheria, and the same preparation was also recommended as a gargle.

Also in Balte boils and furuncles were washed with a flower and leaf decoction, or this same mixture was given as a drink for the same ailments.

In Litin a tincture or infusion was known to cure fever.

In both Korsn and Litin a folk healer placed the steamed flowers and roots topically on areas affected by erysipelas, abscesses, and wounds.

Echoing the ancients' application of the plant for women's medicine, a midwife in Lachovitz made a decoction to be drunk for gynecological conditions such as uterus inflammation; in Makhnivke and Savran midwives used the same brew to treat leucorrhea; and in Khmelnik it was taken to stop menstruation.

For children who suffered from scrofula, folk healers in both Letichev and Broslev gave them a decoction of the plant's flowers.

In Lyubashivka children with convulsions were bathed in a decoction of the plant's flowers by an opshrekherin there (see afterword, p. 255).

And in Jewish communities in Galicia, in the Pale of Settlement, the herb was so well-known and relied on for treating cold symptoms that a pun on the plant's name, *Eibeschte,* was often invoked by Ashkenazi children when someone became sick and required marshmallow tea. In Yiddish God is known as "*der Eiberste*" (the Supreme One), pronounced as *Eibeschte.* In Yiddish this sounds almost exactly like the word for mallow tea (*Eibischtee*), so the person who is a little sick was told that *Eibeschte* would help them.[264]

13

LEPIDIUM RUDERALE

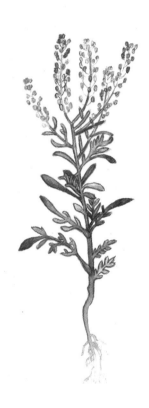

FAMILY: Brassicaceae

COMMON ENGLISH NAMES: narrow-leaf pepperwort, pepperwort, roadside pepperweed, peppergrass

YIDDISH: קרעס ,פֿעפֿערגראָז

HEBREW: שחלים

UKRAINIAN: Вонючка, хріниця вонюча, лихорадочник, вінички, пропасник, зілля від трясці, трава од лихорадки, перчик, цапове зілля, чортове зілля, заячі вінички, слідочки цапові, нечуйвітер, гречечка, вонюче зілля, червишник, бродка, нехворощ польова, курячий поміт

GERMAN: Schutt-Kresse, Stink-Kresse

POLISH: Pieprzyca gruzowa, kłopownyk, metelysznyk, woniuczka, woniucze zileczko

RUSSIAN: Клоповник мусорный

LITHUANIAN: Paprastoji pipirnė

DESCRIPTION AND LOCATION: Biennial native to temperate Asia and northern and Eastern Europe and naturalized in southwestern Europe and North America. Grows from four to eight inches with an erect, nearly smooth stem, branching profusely from its base. Leaves are alternate, also almost without hairs. Lower leaves are narrowly lobed with toothed margins; upper leaves less so. Flowers are symmetrical, commonly slightly reddish, and very small, approximately .04 inches long. Entire plant gives off strong fragrance.[265]

***LEPIDIUM RUDERALE* EARLY REMEDIES:** *Lepidium ruderale* is not a plant often mentioned in most herbal folk remedies. Two related species were known in ancient Greece, *Lepidium latifolium* (pepperwort) and *Lepidium sativum* (garden cress). *Lepidium latifolium* was "a familiar little herb" to the ancient Greeks, and it was preserved in brine and milk to be applied as a plaster for those suffering from diseases of the hip or spleen or sometimes even leprosy. Suspended from the neck, the plant was believed to relieve toothache.[266]

The seed or leaves of *Lepidium sativum*, or garden cress, were known by the ancient Greeks to address similar concerns but also had more varied applications, including expelling intestinal worms, reducing swelling in the spleen, and as an emmenagogue and abortifacient. Combined with other substances, garden cress was of use in cases of impetigo, chest congestions, and as an antidote for snakebites. Burned as a fumigant, it repelled snakes, could curb hair loss, and cause a carbuncle to come to a head.[267]

A thousand years later in the Islamic world, Maimonides also mentioned two similar herbs in his works on plant medicine. Contemporary scholars have tried to disentangle which plants the physician was referring to and have pointed to garden cress, the seeds of which were used in Maimonides's time internally as a diuretic and externally as a cataplasm, or poultice, applied to scrofulous ulcers. The other related plant Maimonides noted, *sitarag*, has been correlated by modern scholars as the Greek pepperwort, or *Lepidium latifolium*. The focus of their research, however, was not the herb's medicinal possibilities but its etymology, tracing the origins of its Arabic name *sitarag* back to the Indian plant name *citrag* by way of Persia.[268]

While scholars' convoluted taxonomy doesn't address the plant's healing qualities, it does serve to illustrate just how complex is the study of herbalism as it crosses historic, geographic, and linguistic boundaries.

By the seventeenth century the only known recorded use of the herb in British folk medicine was that of John Parkinson, who wrote of *L. latifolium*, or "dittander," as it was called, as an additive to ale for laboring women to ensure a speedy delivery.[269]

LEPIDIUM CONTEMPORARY ACTIONS: (some Lepidium species) digestive, circulatory, nutritive, vulnerary, diuretic, detoxifier, cardioprotective, cholagogue, decongestant, hepatic, galactagogue, emmenagogue, aphrodisiac, antibacterial, antioxidant*

LEPIDIUM RUDERALE CONTEMPORARY MEDICINAL PARTS: whole plant

LEPIDIUM RUDERALE IN CONTEMPORARY HERBALISM: In twentieth-century Britain *Lepidium sativum*, when picked before its flavor was strong, contributed "piquancy to salads, garnishes and sauces" as a cut herb. And while the plant has been recognized for containing a natural antibiotic, it has not been in use medicinally.[270]

In contemporary American herbalism the closest documented usage of the *Lepidium* genus is maca, *Lepidium meyenii*. Sometimes known as Peruvian

---

* It's interesting that *L. ruderale* is so widely attested in the towns and villages of the Pale between the wars, while attracting far less overall attention than other species of *Lepidium*. We have grouped comparisons under the broader term.

ginseng, maca is an edible herbaceous biennial of the Brassicaceae family, related to *L. sativum* and *L. campestre*. Maca is native to Peru and has been harvested and used by humans in the puna grasslands of the Andes for centuries as both food and medicine. In the United States contemporary herbalists find the powdered root to be warming and nourishing and a rejuvenating tonic for reproductive health in both men and women. While it has adaptogenic properties, practitioners warn of the plant's ability to mildly inhibit thyroid function if there is a concurrent iodine deficiency.[271]

In the Far East "Semen Lepidii seu Descurainiae," or the dried seeds of *Lepidium apetalum*, have been studied for their anti-inflammatory properties in lung disease as recently as 2019.[272] But this age-old TCM remedy has long been in use as an expectorant, diuretic, anti-inflammatory, sedative, and bronchitis reliever.[273] Colloquially known as pepperweed, the plant is grown in most parts of China, where it is collected in the summer and used unprepared or lightly fried. The seed is broken into pieces before it is prepared as medicine. It has a bitter and pungent flavor and is known to have a very cold property, which assists in its application for removing lung heat and resolving phlegm.[274]

LEPIDIUM RUDERALE IN EUROPEAN HERBALISM IN THE EARLY TWEN-TIETH CENTURY: In the 1930s, the writer and botanist Edith Grey Wheelwright mentioned that while several of the Lepidia or pepperworts were found in the flora of the British Isles, they were not considered indigenous there. Wheelwright characterized the herb as an "insignificant wilding," which gives an indication as to its stature at that time in Britain.[275] Maude Grieve's *A Modern Herbal* doesn't even mention the genus Lepidium whatsoever in her two-volume compendium.

In North America *Lepidium nitidum*, or shining peppergrass, can be found in open places and alkaline soils from Baja California to Washington and Nevada. It was known to the Cahuilla Indians, who cleansed their scalps and prevented baldness with a wash made from the plant's leaves. Incredibly this application echoes the exact remedy Dioscorides noted on the other side of the globe two millennia earlier. The Kumeyaay, formerly known as the Diegueño, found the seeds of the herb helpful with indigestion. For other tribes shining peppergrass offered a vitamin source or helped speed the healing of poison oak rashes. Native peoples in the west also were familiar with other species of the herb such as *L. densiflorum*, to which the Keres turned for headaches, kidney issues, and sunburns. *Lepidium monatum*, or mountain pepperweed, was a Navajo remedy for biliousness and stomach issues, dizziness, and palpitations.[276]

In Russian folk medicine, preparations from *Lepidium ruderale* were used against scurvy and malaria.[277]

LEPIDIUM RUDERALE IN ASHKENAZI HERBALISM IN THE PALE IN THE EARLY TWENTIETH CENTURY:[278] In the Soviet Union between the two world wars, *Lepidium ruderale* was only used in folk medicine and not recognized by official state medicine.

In Maryupol the young plant, pickled, was found to be a remedy for heart trouble. This preference for the plant before it attained a more pungent flavor, not to mention the pickling aspect, recalls the remedies of the ancients who preserved the plant in brine.

A plant decoction or infusion was a remedy for treating malaria in Barditchev, Kolenivka, Letichev, Zvenigorodka, Balte, Birzula, Cherkoss, and Bohslov and for diarrhea and bloody diarrhea in Cherkoss.

As a wash for malarial patients, a decoction or infusion of the plant was given in Korsn.

In Tchan a folk healer burned the dried herb to treat a malarial patient with its smoke. This remedy seems also to recall the ancients who rid themselves of snakes or carbuncles by fumigating affected areas with this plant.

14
MYRISTICA FRAGRANS

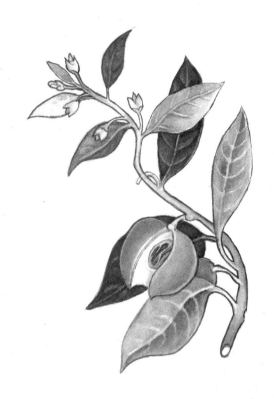

FAMILY: Myristicaceae

COMMON ENGLISH NAMES: nutmeg

YIDDISH: מושקעטבוים

HEBREW: מושקאט

UKRAINIAN: Мускатний горіх

GERMAN: Muskatnuss

POLISH: Gałka muszkatołowa, muszkatołowiec korzenny, muszkatowiec, muszkat

RUSSIAN: Мускатный орех

LITHUANIAN: Kvapusis muskatmedis

DESCRIPTION AND LOCATION: The nutmeg is a tropical evergreen tree that can reach a height of up to fifty feet. It is native to the Moluccan Islands of Indonesia; since being introduced to the European spice trade in the early sixteenth century, it has been cultivated in the West Indies, South Africa, and other tropical regions. Nutmeg trees do not bloom until they are nine years old, at which time the tree begins to fruit and continues to do so without attention for approximately seventy-five years.[279]

The brown wrinkled oval fruit, the size of a marble, contains a kernel that is covered by a bright red membrane. This membrane is known as the spice *mace*, and the kernel it covers as the herb *nutmeg*.[280]

MYRISTICA FRAGRANS EARLY REMEDIES: Historians have made claims that nutmeg was known in the West by the ancients, and Dioscorides himself wrote about a plant called *Holarrhena antidysenterica*, thought to be mace and that some have identified as nutmeg. However, the earliest definitive attested introduction of any kind of plants native to the Moluccan Islands (including the plant called caryophyllorum, a type of carnation) in the West was in the late Roman Empire, in the early fourth century. Many of the nuts found in the region were often described as "musky," which may be the origin of later European names for nutmeg including the French *muscadier,* the German *Muskatnuss,* the Italian *noce moscata,* and the Spanish *nuez moscada.*[281] By the ninth and tenth centuries Arab physicians attested to the herb.[282] A hundred years later, Maimonides recorded several of the plant's names in Arabic, one of which translates into English as "the aromatic nut."[283]

The first writer in the West to document nutmeg was Simeon Seth, most likely a doctor of Eastern origin, possibly from Persia or the Arab world, who in 1078 referred to the plant in Greek as *Karyon aromatikon.* Two decades later

Constantinus Africanus, a physician living in Salerno, distinguished between nutmeg and mace, thus separating the two individual substances and contributing the first use of both names in European cultural history.[284] At the beginning of the twelfth century, Nicolaus Praepositus further distinguished between nutmeg and mace in his *Antidotarium*, a compendium of medicinal plant recipes.

By the mid-twelfth century it appears nutmeg had begun to acquire a wider reputation. In 1150 the German abbess and herbalist Hildegard was familiar enough with the herb to characterize the spice nutmeg as strong with great warmth and good temperament, opening the heart of anyone who consumed it, thereby promoting good disposition. To quell noxious humors, she recommended a paste made of nutmeg and cinnamon to calm all the bitterness of the heart and mind to make one joyful.[285] For a serious lung disorder she further recommended a galangal, fennel, nutmeg, and feverfew preparation to be taken daily on an empty stomach, so that their combined odor would enter into the lungs and suppress foul breath.[286]

The abbess's reliance on nutmeg to open one's heart to promote a good disposition via its action through the lungs is fascinating in its parallel to the TCM philosophy of lung health's association with the emotion of grief. In TCM it is understood that if someone suffers from respiratory ailments, underlying grief may be the cause. The connection between these two functions, breathing and emotion, is a recurring theme in Hildegard's work. And as if to underscore her recommendations, a contemporary laboratory study demonstrates nutmeg also possesses antidepressant qualities in addition to its other virtues.[287]

Written evidence in other parts of the continent, at roughly the same time that Hildegard flourished, indicates that by 1158 the city of Genoa imported ten pounds of nutmeg from Alexandria. While the herb was a relatively rare article imported into Europe, it is obvious that both nutmeg and mace were used not only as healing remedies on the Continent but also for festive occasions. In a poem by Petrus de Ebulo, Roman streets are described as being scented with a combination of balsam, frankincense, aloe, nutmeg, cinnamon, and nardus during the coronation of the Emperor Heinrich in 1191.

By the thirteenth century the record indicates increasing quantities of the herb were entering Europe. In 1228 written evidence shows nutmeg not only in Italy but also in Marseilles, and by 1259 in Germany as well.

Pharmacological knowledge was increasing by the late twelfth century among the Byzantines in Asia Minor too, presumably because more exotic imports were traded directly with the Arabs. By the end of the century Actuarius, the physician at the court of Constantinople, referred to an oily nut called *myristica* and recommended it be used, along with other roots and flowers such as violet, rosemary, and rose, as an antidote called *dianthon*. Albertus Magnus, a German friar and alchemist in the thirteenth century, also documents knowledge of the herb.[288]

Paracelsus, in his sixteenth-century alchemical writings, described the aromatic nut but only addressed its outer covering, mace, and its strengthening powers.[289]

When Tobias ha-Kohen wrote his text in the eighteenth century, he referred to *muskato* several times. Sexual concerns, diarrhea and constipation, and oral health are some of the conditions addressed therein with various related preparations of the herb.[290]

MYRISTICA FRAGRANS **CONTEMPORARY ACTIONS:** (Western) carminative, culinary spice, anti-nausea; (Eastern) aromatic, astringent, circulatory stimulant, aphrodisiac, rubefacient, sedative, nervine, appetite stimulant

MYRISTICA FRAGRANS **CONTEMPORARY MEDICINAL PARTS:** nut-like seed, without red mace covering

MYRISTICA FRAGRANS **IN CONTEMPORARY HERBALISM:** "It is said that on the islands where the nutmeg grows, the aroma is so powerful the birds of the air become intoxicated with the scent," wrote early twentieth-century British herbalist Hilda Leyel, whose pen name was Mrs. C. F. Leyel.[291] Humans too have appreciated the delicate qualities of the nutmeg, but its journey to our kitchen spice racks has been a circuitous one.

In its native terrain, and particularly in India, nutmeg has always been relied on for its special medicinal powers in Ayurvedic medicine. The plant is mainly taken to relieve insomnia; it's the freshly dried plant, immediately encapsulated, that retains the best healing properties. Because nutmeg's sedating action has a predictable delay of three and a half to five hours to take effect after ingesting, other herbs, such as poppy, are recommended as part of a more complex formula to bring on sleep at the outset so that a full eight hours of rest will be guaranteed.

In addition to nutmeg's soporific properties, in Ayurvedic medicine the herb is also considered a mild aphrodisiac; however, its more potent sedative qualities necessitate that nutmeg be a relatively minor ingredient in these preparations. Its moderately drying (astringent and diuretic) action, which can cause constipation, makes it useful for helping clear up diarrhea, especially in children. As a carminative, nutmeg is considered by Ayurvedic medicine to be similar in action to cinnamon and clove. Nutmeg is also included in formulas for hemorrhoids and can be applied topically as a paste by adding a solid fat. A butter made from the herb is an ingredient in ointments used for joint pain such as arthritis. Nutmeg's other Ayurvedic actions include hepatoprotective, anti-catarrhal, and respiratory soothing for cough and congestion.[292]

Generally speaking, in the West nutmeg is not much used medicinally in contemporary herbalism; rather, it is considered an aromatic spice.[293] But in the early 1970s American herbalists and others were adding the kernel's oil as a scent for soaps and perfumes or recommending the herb as a carminative. An ointment made from pressed nutmeg and mace was found to be a counterirritant in the treatment of arthritis, and as part of a more complex formula, the herb was also included in a recipe for tooth powder.[294]

Around roughly the same period, German herbalists were incorporating nutmeg as an ingredient in homemade nonalcoholic beverages.[295]

MYRISTICA FRAGRANS IN EUROPEAN HERBALISM IN THE EARLY TWEN-TIETH CENTURY: By the early decades of the twentieth century, nutmeg was still a rare commodity that tempted its purveyors to adulterate their product, thereby selling unsuspecting customers an inferior substance. Oil of nutmeg was used to hide the taste of various drugs or as a local stimulant to the gastrointestinal tract, while the powdered herb was rarely given alone but rather was an ingredient in a number of medicines. In Britain the medicinal properties of nutmeg and mace were described as identical, and both were used as a carminative and an antinausea and were mixed with lard to relieve hemorrhoids. It was also noted that as an addition to drinks the herb was agreeable to convalescents; others roasted the nut and then applied it internally as a remedy for leucorrhea.[296]

The expressed oil was also once an ingredient of the *Emplastrum picis*, a rubefacient plaster, used for catarrhal complaints of the chest, chronic inflammation of the liver, and rheumatic pain of the joints and muscles.[297]

In the Ruhr district of Germany at the turn of the twentieth century, when a child had diarrhea, their food was sprinkled with nutmeg to aid in digestion. In western Bohemia, to aid digestion, toasted bread with nutmeg dipped in wine was put in a sack and placed directly on the navel. And for a child with diarrhea, a plaster made of bread crusts, juniper berries, caraway seeds, ginger, cinnamon, cloves, and nutmeg was applied to the belly. There they also took a mixture of finely chopped nutmeg or garlic in brandy for abdominal pain. The Slovaks gave adult patients with diarrhea a combination of nutmeg, camphor, opium, black pepper, gall apples, and ginger.[298]

Aside from the remark about convalescents, the only clue in the West of nutmeg's ability to curb insomnia comes from Leyel, who mentioned the herb's presence as a conceit of an earlier generation: "the silver graters our grandmothers wore on their chatelaines" were used to make nutmeg tea, which "supposedly had restorative powers."[299] She also documented a recipe for quelling insomnia:

> Grate 3 ounces of nutmeg. Put into a quart bottle and fill up with good brandy. Cork and shake every day for a fortnight, then pour off without disturbing the sediment. 3 or 4 drops will flavour a pint of liquid. To help the sleepless: 10 drops in a glass of hot water or milk. The dose can be repeated after 2 hours.[300]

All sources advise caution when using this herb and that larger doses of nutmeg are narcotic and produce dangerous symptoms.

MYRISTICA FRAGRANS IN ASHKENAZI HERBALISM IN THE PALE IN THE EARLY TWENTIETH CENTURY: In Pauline Wengeroff's autobiography of her life in the Pale of Settlement, *Memoirs of a Grandmother,* she recalls the relationship she had with her husband's grandmother, Beile. The extended family at that time, in the mid-to-late nineteenth century, lived in Konotip (present-day Konotop, Ukraine), which is slightly north of and halfway between present-day Kiev and Kharkov. Beile was Konotip's midwife and also a very well-respected member of her community. After Wengeroff had given birth to the family's first grandson, Beile looked after the new mother and child. When Wengeroff had trouble sleeping, one of the remedies she remembers Beile making for her was a "trianke," a Yiddish word that may have its origins in the Slavic root for three. The trianke was given as a sleep aid and consisted of "cooked honey, which had stood for several days in a warm oven and was poured over a spirits extract of spices like kalhan (galangal, likely *Alpinia officinarum*), badjan (star anise, or *Illicium verum*), nutmeg, cinnamon, clove, figs and carob bean."[301]

What's fascinating about this story—aside from the fact that it is currently the only published memoir of a Jewish woman from the Pale of Settlement—is the author's nonchalant mention of the common use of somewhat exotic herbs and spices in a small town in Eastern Europe. This passage attests to the deep and wide body of healing knowledge from which Ashkenazi folk healers drew to care for their families and, by extension, the larger local populations. In this instance the soporific and relaxing qualities of the foreign herb nutmeg, so long valued and well understood in the East but less known elsewhere, were almost being intuited by a humble midwife in her role as one of the town's traditional healers.

15

NYMPHAEA ALBA

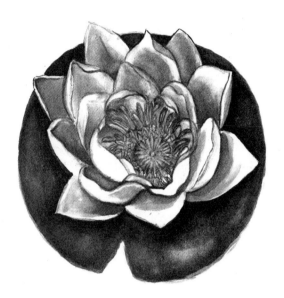

FAMILY: Nymphaeaceae

COMMON ENGLISH NAMES: European white water lily

YIDDISH: וואַסער–ליליע, וואַיסקריגנעלע, שבועות-ראָיז

HEBREW: ליליום אלבו

UKRAINIAN: Латаття біле, латаття, біле жіноче латаття, латач білий, латаки білі, латахи, лотаки жіночі, лататник, момич, момич білий, момич білий жіночий, баньки, баньки білі, біленькі квітки, маківки, маківки білі, сплавник, волові очка, підбіл, водяний корінь

GERMAN: Lilie, Seerose

POLISH: Grażel żółty, grzybienie białe, nenufar, lilia wodna

RUSSIAN: Кушвинка белая, лилия водяная

LITHUANIAN: Paprastoji vandens lelija

DESCRIPTION AND LOCATION: Native to North Africa, Europe, and temperate and tropical regions of Asia, *Nymphaea alba* is a perennial water plant that prefers large ponds and lakes and grows one to five feet in depth. Circular, floating leaves can be up to a foot in diameter and can range up to six feet from the plant on long thin stems. White, bowl-shaped flowers contain many small yellow stamens and bloom from July to August, yielding seeds that ripen from August to October. The species is hermaphrodite (has both male and female organs) and is pollinated by insects.[302]

NYMPHAEA ALBA **EARLY REMEDIES:** The ancient Greeks named *Nymphaea alba* to honor its preference for watery habitats. Combined with wine, preparations of the plant were imbibed to benefit the colicky and dysenteric and to calm an inflamed spleen. As a plaster the root soothed stomach and bladder pain, cleared "dull-white leprosies" as an infusion, and, when combined with pitch (a resin derived from plants), treated bald spots.

Dioscorides mentions both the seeds and the roots for their reputation as a drink to deter nocturnal emissions. In an interesting aside, many hundreds of years later, Tobias ha-Kohen also documented the plant's utility concerning sexual matters, especially with regard to semen.[303] This particular application in the Ashkenazi Pale of Settlement was probably recommended as a prophylactic against "visits from Lilith," a gender-nonspecific demon who was often blamed for stealing semen from unsuspecting men as they slept.[304] In addition ancient Greek women took the root and seed steeped in red wine as a remedy for leucorrhea.[305]

Maimonides wrote of the many Arabic names for the plant, which can be translated as "young bride" and "tomb of bees." He also noted that in the original Sanskrit *nilotpala* meant "blue lotus," which became transformed into *nenuphar* in French and English. The dried flowers were sold in the bazaars to make compresses that were known to refresh and calm.[306]

In ancient Russia it was known as "grass lump" by peasants who used its roots, petals, and leaves for medicinal purposes. In more shamanistic realms it was believed that the aquatic plant protected against all troubles and misfortunes, witchcraft, and evil spirits. Russian folklore called the water lily "the flower of the mermaids," because the long rhizome resembled a tail, and the white flower a body.

Decoctions of rhizomes of water lilies once were included in the diet of monks to dull their sex drive. To ensure an abundant supply of the anaphrodisiac, monasteries maintained large reservoirs where the plants could grow in profusion.[307]

Avicenna also documented the medicinal qualities of this aqueous plant, describing a tincture of its roots for spleen tumors and a decoction of the seeds or leaves for poorly healing wounds and ulcers.[308]

NYMPHAEA ALBA CONTEMPORARY ACTIONS: *Nymphaea alba*'s medicinal application in contemporary herbalism, at least in the written record, is sparse. As a folk remedy, even in Europe, the plant seems to have fallen out of favor in the last century. Late twentieth-century and early twenty-first-century European sources describe the root as anti-scrofulous, astringent, cardiotonic, demulcent, and sedative.[309]

NYMPHAEA ALBA CONTEMPORARY MEDICINAL PARTS: root or rhizome

NYMPHAEA ALBA IN CONTEMPORARY HERBALISM: Scant information published in the West records that a decoction of the root is used in the treatment of dysentery or diarrhea caused by irritable bowel syndrome. It has also been described as a treatment for chronic bronchitis and kidney pain and as a gargle for a sore throat. For vaginal soreness and discharge, the rhizome can be included in a douche preparation. Additionally a poultice to treat boils and abscesses can be made from the rhizome.

The flowers are anaphrodisiac and sedative with a generally calming effect upon the nervous system and, mirroring the Eastern European monks' usage, can reduce sex drive, which may be helpful for insomnia, anxiety, and similar complaints.[310]

The Russian website *Lektrava* relays the use of white water lilies as a traditional medicine for a wide variety of diseases and also states the plant has long been used by magicians as a love potion.

For medicinal purposes the rhizomes, leaves, and flowers of the plant are used. Rhizomes in the form of a decoction or alcohol tincture are effective as an astringent taken internally. Topically the same decoction is beneficial for rheumatism, for wounds as a hemostatic, for skin inflammation, for astringing diarrhea, for treating cystitis, dysentery, and gonorrhea, and for gynecological problems, in particular leucorrhea. In addition the roots of water lilies can be used like mustard plasters. A broth is drunk for tuberculosis and to increase lactation in nursing women.

The leaves are infused to heal ulcers in the mouth, and externally the same preparation can be used for boils, skin inflammations, dropsy, abscesses, and as an anti-inflammatory for wounds.

A tincture of the leaves and stems is indicated for diseases of the kidneys and bladder and for intestinal ulcers. A decoction of leaves and roots treats liver diseases including hepatitis.

The flowers are used to relieve insomnia, the pain from neuralgia, and rheumatism. They are considered soothing for the nervous system, particularly for treating anxiety and depression. The flowers are also considered antipyretic and emollient. Russians have made decoctions of water lilies to treat seizures and toothache pain. Musicians gargle with a decoction or tincture of seeds to support the vocal cords to strengthen the voice. A decoction of the roots in beer is a remedy for hair loss. Fresh or preserved juice of the plant lightens freckles and other pigmentation. An infusion of the petals of a water lily is added to baths.[311]

NYMPHAEA ALBA **IN HERBALISM IN THE EARLY TWENTIETH CENTURY:** In Brazil in the early twentieth century, *Nymphaea alba* was a common water plant, the rootstocks of which were used as astringent, narcotic, and styptic medicines and for the treatment of dysentery. For ulcers, especially of the stomach, a preparation of the flowers was given. The 1925 *Nueva farmacopea mexicana* also specified the plant's major characteristic as astringent.[312]

In Russian folk medicine, a decoction from the flowers was used as a laxative and against jaundice and insomnia; a decoction from the rhizomes was used to treat diseases of the kidneys and urinary tract, and against intestinal infections, menstrual disorders, and cancer.[313]

A 1941 Russian medicinal plants pamphlet described the aquatic herb as well-known to the population and growing everywhere in European Russia and

Siberia. The dried root, the source noted, was ground into flour because of its high starch content, and the seeds were roasted for a coffee substitute.[314] And Grieve's classic reference, *A Modern Herbal*, makes note of a completely cured case of uterine cancer in the early years of the twentieth century using a decoction of the plant's close relative, *Nymphaea odorata*.[315]

NYMPHAEA ALBA IN ASHKENAZI HERBALISM IN THE PALE IN THE EARLY TWENTIETH CENTURY:[316] While western Europe had for quite some time all but ignored the plant, it is plain the *Nymphaea alba* was much valued in the east. Among Ashkenazim it was used most often in folk medicine in the northern part of the Kamenetz-Podolski region (Pravopobereshe), on the right bank of the Dnieper, home to many Ashkenazi settlements. It was a common aquatic plant there, found in slow streams, ponds, lakes, and rivers.

While the following water lily remedies recorded in the shtetls are more in line with Russian traditions, healers in these towns and villages had their own interpretations of the plant's virtues. In folk medicine, decoctions and tinctures of the roots and flowers were commonly sought, especially as a remedy for the treatment of heart disease, edema of the arms, legs, and eyelids, and shortness of breath in Monasterishtche, Kresilev, Slovita, Olt-Kosntin, Ritzev, Polona, Bobinka, and Balte.

A similar decoction was used by traditional practitioners to treat kidney diseases in Anapol; head colds in Monasterishtche, Broslev, Barditchev, and Bohslov; as a remedy for tuberculosis in Bobinka, Litin, and Birzula; to treat malaria in Ulanov; and to fortify those with anemia and meagerness in Bohslov.

Midwives in Olt-Kosntin, Lachovitz, and Vinitza gave a decoction of dried and powdered rootstocks or a tincture of roots and flowers (or of flowers alone) to women suffering from heavy menstrual flow.

A combined infusion of the flowers of *Nymphaea alba* and *Robinia pseudoacacia* (black locust tree) was used to stop hemorrhages in Bohslov and Vinitza.

A powder prepared from the dried rootstocks and leaves was sprinkled on wounds in the small towns of Ritzev and Polona.

One folk healer in Vinitza prepared an ointment from the water lily's flowers steeped in sunflower oil specifically as a topical for wounds.

A decoction or tincture of rootstocks and flowers (or the flowers and leaves) of *Nymphaea alba* and the rootstocks of *Nuphar luteum* (yellow water lily) was given to those suffering from catarrh of the stomach in Vinitza; in Letichev the same formula was used by folk healers there for dysentery and hemorrhoids.

Immersion in a rootstock decoction bath was a folk remedy for rheumatism in Slovita.

The lily's fresh leaves were applied to burns in Litin.

16

PAEONIA OFFICINALIS

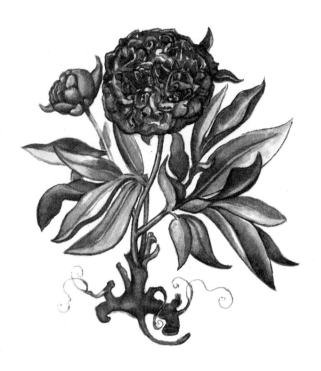

FAMILY: Paeoniaceae

COMMON ENGLISH NAMES: common peony, garden peony

YIDDISH: פּעאָן, פּיװאָניע

HEBREW: פיאוניאה, ארמונית

UKRAINIAN: Півонія лікарська, півонія, червона півонія, певонія, біла певонія, пивонія, павонія, півник, піон

GERMAN: Pfingstrose

POLISH: Piwonia lekarska

RUSSIAN: Пион лекарственный

LITHUANIAN: Vaistinis bijūnas

DESCRIPTION AND LOCATION: Perennial native to France, Switzerland, and Italy that grows wild in southern Europe and cultivated elsewhere in gardens. Thick knobby rootstocks produce a green fleshy stem that can reach from two to three feet in height. Leaves have three or six oval-shaped leaflets. Large single red or purplish rose-like flowers bloom from May to August.[317]

***PAEONIA OFFICINALIS* EARLY REMEDIES:** The genus is alleged to have been named for the physician Paeos, who, with the aid of this plant, cured the wounds suffered by Pluto and other gods during the Trojan War.

Many superstitions are connected with the peony. In ancient times it was thought to be of divine origin, emanating from the moon at night, and therefore believed to protect shepherds, their flocks, and harvests from injury, to repel evil spirits, and to avert storms.[318]

Pliny the Elder wrote that peony, in addition to its other virtues, "also prevents the mocking delusions that the Fauns bring on us in our sleep."[319]

Dioscorides described the plant in great detail and singled out the root for medicinal powers. It was taken for stomachaches, jaundice, urinary system complaints, to stop diarrhea, and to "avert . . . stones when children drink and eat." A quantity of fifteen seeds taken with a hydromel or wine was believed to alleviate the gasping experienced during nightmares, because in ancient times it was thought that bad dreams were caused by demons who strangled their slumbering victims.

Preparations of peony were also taken for gynecological applications. It was "given to women who are not cleansed after giving birth," and also it was known to draw "down the menses when a quantity the size of an almond" was drunk. "Uterine suffocation" (a belief held by the ancient Greek physicians regarding the uterus's role in gynecological ailments and a term that has had many interpretations over the centuries) and uterine pains were also treated with peony.[320]

The German abbess and herbalist Hildegard recommended the fiery strength of "*beonia*" as a treatment for tertian and quartan fevers, both today associated with the intermittent fevers of malaria. For these she prescribed the pounded root in wine or pulverized in flour and mixed with lard or poppy seed oil into a paste that was to be eaten often. The seed, dipped in honey and placed on the tongue, could bring a deranged person back to their senses. For phlegm in the head and chest, excessive mucus, or bad breath, the transversely cut root mixed with the plant's seed and boiled in wine was to be drunk warm and often to purge the head and chest and eliminate halitosis. For those with the falling sickness, as epilepsy was formerly known, peony seed that was dipped in the blood of a swallow then rolled immediately in flour and put in the mouth was said to cure the condition. For worms destroying one's hair, a lye made with peony seed and root washed the parasites away. Peony leaves and roots placed in one's clothing were also said to deter pests from ruining one's wardrobe.[321]

The Sephardic physician Maimonides around the same period identified the plant as *fawaniya* ("peony"), *du al-hams habbat*, "the one with five seeds," from the Greek *pentorobon*, and also *ward al-hamir*, or "donkey rose." In Egypt and Syria it was known as *ud as-salib* ("wood of the cross"), and in the bazaars of Cairo, the roots of peony were sold in thick fragments that were added to beverages as an antispasmodic. At one time they were used against epilepsy, "by promenading the root fragments attached in the form of a cross over the chest." This remedy was still in use by some Christian communities in the Near East at the end of the nineteenth century.[322]

In medieval Europe it was a custom to wear a chain of beads cut from peony roots as a protection against all sorts of illness and injury, to assist children in teething, and as a remedy for insanity. The Native people of North America used a tea made from the roots for lung troubles.[323]

Sixteenth-century Polish poet Mikołaj Rej declared peonies were second only to roses in orchards and gardens.[324]

When the physician Tobias ha-Kohen wrote his medical text, he invoked the peony for a number of treatments including as both a protection against fear, and he recommended it mixed with other herbs such as *Acorus calamus* (calamus), *Verbena* sp. (verbena), *Artemisia abrotanum* (southern wormwood), and *Marrubium vulgare* (horehound) to cleanse the head.[325]

PAEONIA OFFICINALIS **CONTEMPORARY ACTIONS:** antispasmodic, diuretic, sedative

PAEONIA OFFICINALIS **CONTEMPORARY MEDICINAL PARTS:** rootstock, dried

PAEONIA OFFICINALIS **IN CONTEMPORARY HERBALISM:** In the 1970s American herbalists described peony as an old remedy for jaundice and for ailments of the urinary system using an extract made by steeping the root in wine. A decoction of the root was also known to treat gout, asthma with cramps, and (in very small doses) eclampsia. It was warned, however, that the entire plant is poisonous, the flowers especially so, and even a tea made from the flowers can be fatal—and in fact, the plant should not be used at all unless under strict medical supervision.[326]

In TCM two species of peony are used. The tree peony—formerly classed as *Paeonia Moutan* and now considered part of a group of cultivars grown for thousands of years in China and known in the west collectively as *Paeonia suffruticosa*—is valued for the healing properties found in the skin of its root. Its cooling properties and its affinity for the heart and liver are employed.[327] *P. suffruticosa* is considered a pungent and antibacterial circulatory stimulant that can lower blood pressure with anti-inflammatory, analgesic, sedative actions. Known in China as *mu dan pi*, tree peony is used to cool the blood and has also been applied in a childhood eczema project in London. Decoctions of the root in combination with other herbs are used for feverish conditions like nosebleeds or for hot, dry conditions like eczema or liver disharmonies. The root bark is also considered a good antiseptic for boils and abscesses.[328]

The red- or white-flowered *Paeonia lactiflora* is characterized as sour, bitter, and cold with actions that include antibacterial, antispasmodic, anti-inflammatory, analgesic, tranquilizing, and blood-pressure lowering. The root of the white peony, known in China as *bai shao yao*, nourishes the blood rather than cooling it and is considered one of the great gynecological tonics, used often in menstrual disorders. It has a much more specific action on the liver than red peony, soothing it and improving the organ's function.

The root of red *P. lactiflora*, known as *chi shao yao* in China, is considered cooling to the blood, to move stagnating blood and relieve pain. A decoction of the root is given for conditions involving overheated blood, certain types of eczema, skin inflammations, nosebleeds, and pain connected with injury. In the 1990s experiments in England combined red peony root and other Chinese herbs to successfully treat childhood eczema.[329]

Contemporary American clinical herbalists recognize *P. lactiflora*'s actions as an alterative, analgesic, anti-inflammatory, and antispasmodic, and they recommend the herb as a decoction or tincture for amenorrhea, for its ability to move and build blood, soothe abdominal pain, and cool hot flashes and night sweats.[330]

In his text on medical herbalism, renowned herbalist David Hoffmann noted that *P. suffruticosa*, while part of a list regarding pregnancy warnings in the *Botanical Safety Handbook*, included no clarification as to whether its dangers were based on actual clinical trials or merely theoretical extrapolations from in vitro studies on the plant's constituents, thus limiting the source's usefulness for those inquiring on the plant's medicine.[331]

In North America the western peony, or *Paeonia brownii*, grows on open dry mountain slopes, scrublands, and sagebrush. Indigenous peoples have used a root tea as a remedy for "nausea, stomach ache, indigestion, constipation, diarrhea, coughs, sore throat, colds, pneumonia, tuberculosis, heart trouble, chest pains, kidney problems, venereal disease, and sore eyes; also to fatten people and horses and as a wash to relieve headache." The root was powdered and poulticed on skin abrasions. Crushed roots treated boils or deep wounds. A related species, *P. californica*, was eaten to quell indigestion by the Kumeyaay peoples also known as Tipai-Ipai, Kamia, or Diegueño.[332]

PAEONIA OFFICINALIS IN EUROPEAN HERBALISM IN THE EARLY TWENTIETH CENTURY: In early twentieth-century England, *Paeonia officinalis* was considered antispasmodic, and the use of its root was recorded as having been successful in the quelling of convulsions and spasmodic nervous conditions such as epilepsy. It had also been considered effective for curing lunacy.[333]

In other parts of Europe, the seeds of "the gout rose" were used in children's dentistry. Seeds and roots were hung around the neck to protect against epileptic episodes, blood stagnation in women, and as a remedy for asthma and rheumatism.[334]

In Russia the peony was used as a remedy for epilepsy and colic in children. Its rootstocks had laxative properties that were known among the peasants as a stomach remedy and used in powder form for diarrhea and stomachache. It was also used in Soviet veterinary medicine.[335]

In Russia *Paeonia anomala* (a related plant that does not grow in the Pale) was used in folk medicine for the following: carcinomas of the liver, stomach, and intestines, postpartum uterine atony, tuberculosis, epilepsy, malaria, gout, rheumatism, coughs, and functional disorders of the nervous system. The plant was also used as an abortifacient and galactagogue, and in the Krasnodar region for liver, stomach, and uterine malignancies.[336]

PAEONIA OFFICINALIS IN ASHKENAZI HERBALISM IN THE PALE IN THE EARLY TWENTIETH CENTURY:[337] Peony is referred to in the Soviet-era report on folk medicine in the Pale as a collective species, and, unlike other plants in the study, was reported to have been used almost exclusively for gynecological diseases in the towns and villages surveyed.

As a remedy for epilepsy, an infusion of the flowers was taken in Lachovitz.

As a remedy for leucorrhea, a midwife in Olt-Kosntin reported an infusion of peony's flower was given.

In Kresilev, Tchan, Anapol, Barditchev, Ulanov, Kanev, Cherkoss, Zvenigorodka, and Balte, a flower decoction or infusion was taken by women in order to induce menstruation. In Balte a root decoction was also reported for this use.

17

PLANTAGO MAJOR

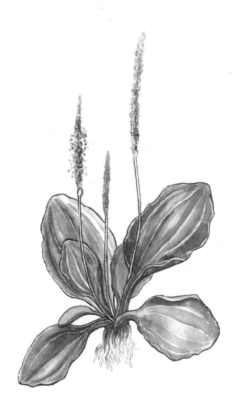

FAMILY: Plantaginaceae

COMMON ENGLISH NAMES: broad-leaved plantain, ripple grass, waybread, waybroad, snakeweed, cuckoo's bread, Englishman's foot, white man's foot, St. Patrick's leaf

YIDDISH: וועגבלאַט, וועגשפּרייטער, באָפקע

HEBREW: לחך

UKRAINIAN: Подорожник великий, подорожник, бабка, бабки, свинжильник

GERMAN: Wegerich

POLISH: Babka zwyczajna, babka większa, babka lancetowata

RUSSIAN: Подорожник большой

LITHUANIAN: Plačialapis gyslotis

DESCRIPTION AND LOCATION: Perennial plant arising from a rosette of ribbed leaves and producing wind-pollinated flowers on erect stalks.[338] Found in meadows, roadsides, agricultural lands, and most everywhere inhabited by humans. Native to Europe and naturalized in the Eastern and Pacific coastal regions of the US and Canada.[339]

PLANTAGO MAJOR **EARLY REMEDIES:** *Plantago* has a long and illustrious herbal history. The Anglo-Saxon name for plantain was *waybroed* or *waybrode*, later becoming *waybread* because of its preference for growing by the way or path, not its prospect as a food.[340]

Much as today, the ancient Greeks were familiar with two types, the leaves of which were known to have astringent properties that made excellent poultices for treating many malignancies including elephantiasis, sores, hemorrhages, ulcers, carbuncles, shingles and pustules, dog bites, burns, and a variety of inflammations. Athenian healers prescribed the leaves boiled with salt and vinegar for those suffering from dysentery or colic, or they made a meal-like paste for treating edema, asthma, or epilepsy. In addition the juice from the leaves acted as a mouthwash to clear ulcers and bleeding gums, or, mixed with Cimolian earth or white lead, could cure erysipelas. The ancients also found it beneficial for earaches and in treating ailments of the eyes. For tuberculosis or dysentery, it was prepared as a clyster, or enema. In gynecological matters, when applied on a wad of wool, it was given as a pessary for "uterine suffocation" or discharges. The plant's seed was drunk with wine to stop diarrhea and the spitting of blood. The root, chewed or decocted, could stop toothaches. Both the leaves and root were taken with grape syrup for bladder and kidney ailments. Fevers were helped by the root as well, and some people were even known to wear the roots as amulets to discourage scrofulous swellings of the glands.[341] Galen was succinct with his recommendations and called for the leaves to be pulped with bread and applied as an astringent.[342]

A thousand years on, Maimonides noted that in Arabic plantain is called the "dog's tongue" and the "rat's tail," and that it was also referred to as "cold and peaceful." Druggists of Cairo sold two types: the seed of one served as an astringent, while the leaves of the other were recommended for cataplasms, or poultices.[343]

The German abbess Hildegard regarded the plantain as part of an antidote for poisons to be used with magical words to bring health, strength, and good fortune to those that carried it with them.[344] *Wegerich*, as it was called in German, was known to her as both warm and dry. It treated gout, soothed a cramp in the side, and sped the healing of an insect bite; it was also connected with mending broken bones and for purging oneself after taking a love potion.[345] Could it be that Shakespeare mentioned plantain twice as a healer of broken shins because he had read or knew of the abbess's work some four centuries before his own?[346]

By the time Tobias ha-Kohen wrote of the plant, he associated its use with skin ailments, kidney and urine concerns, and digestion.[347]

A bit later in Switzerland, Samuel-Auguste Tissot wrote of the plant's connection in treating dysentery and for the bite of a mad dog when mixed as a powder with several other dessicated and pulverized herbs.[348]

By the early nineteenth century the Bavarian priest Sebastian Kneipp praised the herb, writing that "plantain closes the gaping wound with a seam of gold thread; for just as gold will not admit of rust, so the plantain will not admit of rotting and gangrenous flesh."[349]

PLANTAGO MAJOR **CONTEMPORARY ACTIONS:** antiseptic, antivenomous, astringent, decongestant, demulcent, drawing, emollient, vulnerary, anti-inflammatory, antimicrobial

PLANTAGO MAJOR **CONTEMPORARY MEDICINAL PARTS:** leaves, seeds

PLANTAGO MAJOR **IN CONTEMPORARY HERBALISM:** The humble plantain, the plant most people literally step right over without the slightest notice, has long been a favorite remedy of American herbalists. One modern recipe calls for the juice of the plant to be mixed with the oil of roses and applied to the temples to ease headache, or to the hands and feet for alleviating the pain from gout and arthritis. A decoction can be applied topically to heal scabs and itches, ringworm, shingles sores, and bruises. Hemorrhoid sufferers find relief with mashed leaf applications. In addition one preparation has been employed as a douche for leucorrhea, another for diarrhea, coughs, colds, and bronchitis,[350] a diuretic, an alterative, a promoter of fertility, a counterirritant for nettles, a styptic, a toothache soother, and a laxative.[351] Gastrointestinal ailments and worms can also be voided by taking the fresh juice from the whole plant. One herbalist from the 1970s added that common plantain is sometimes recommended to increase virility, and they proposed that the remedy may have been influenced by the bloom's suggestive flower spike shape.[352] My own experience with plantain is as a quick "spit poultice" for mosquito or spider bites; the itch disappears almost as soon as the plant touches the affected area.

In twenty-first-century herbalism of the West, plantain's reputation as a safe primary topical healing agent is well-known.[353] Powdered, the leaves can be added to food or used as an herbal first aid sprinkled on infections. As an internal remedy, a mild flavored tea can be made from the leaves to treat liver sluggishness and inflammations of the digestive tract. The seeds from a *Plantago* species, rich in mucilage, are the main ingredient in commercial laxative preparations.[354]

When paired with *Grindelia squarrosa* (gumweed), plantain helps draw out sticky phlegm with its cooling, moistening, and astringing properties.[355] British herbalists also share this reliance on plantain's demulcent properties when treating respiratory complaints.[356]

Other contemporary British herbalists find plantain preferable to dock leaf for nettle stings and its antihistamine effect beneficial for hayfever and other allergies when combined as a tea with elderflower and mint. For painful shins after a radiation burn, one herbalist found success by mixing plantain juice with slippery elm powder.[357]

In folk medicine of the British Isles, plantain has primarily been used to stop bleeding, and "has been used in inflammation of the skin, malignant ulcers, intermittent fever, etc., and as a vulnerary, and externally as a stimulant application to sores."[358] Other uses recorded have been for the healing of rashes and burns, the prevention of festering wounds, to treat varicosities, to draw the pus out of an infection, to soothe stings, and as a tonic mixed with *Achillea millefolium* (yarrow) and *Urtica dioica* (nettles).

In Ireland some believe that one side of the plantain's leaf draws out the toxin from a wound and the other side does the healing. There the juice is drunk for coughs, liver trouble, and jaundice; for children who are deemed delicate, the juice is given mixed with milk. Records show the plant has also been used to soothe sore eyes, a treatment that recalls the ancient Greeks.[359]

Older country women practicing folk medicine in Poland have long relied on the healing properties of the plantain's fresh leaves for treating skin ailments in both humans and animals. At times the crushed leaves are mixed with lard or bread and then applied as a poultice to ulcers or boils. The leaves are also juiced to treat bee stings, fevers, respiratory complaints, tuberculosis, internal bleeding, and rheumatism, to soothe mucous membranes, and to cleanse the blood. Fresh roots are placed in the ear for toothaches and removed once they become blackened.[360]

After long being considered a weed, plantain is now cultivated in Russia for pharmaceutical use. In folk medicine the fresh juice or a crushed leaf poultice is used topically to treat cuts, burns, wounds, ulcers, and insect stings as well as snakebites.

Country people still use these old methods when emergency medical treatment is not immediately available. Headache and respiratory complaints can be soothed with an infusion of plantain, or as a gargle it's used to relieve toothache. In official medicine the fresh juice from the leaves is recommended for gastrointestinal ailments including gastritis and stomach and duodenal ulcers, for improving appetite, and regulating stomach acidity.

The juice of fresh plantain leaves is prescribed by official Russian medicine practitioners to treat chronic gastritis and gastrointestinal ulcers, to relieve stomach pain, improve appetite, and increase the acidity of the gastric juices. When powdered, the seeds can have a purgative effect and are prescribed as an astringent for diarrhea when it occurs as a side effect of tuberculosis. In the 1960s Soviet Union, a commercial plantain preparation was sold throughout the country to treat stomach concerns.[361]

Lithuanian application of plantain parallels that of modern Russia with two additional uses: as a treatment for atherosclerosis, and the herb's young fresh leaves are added to salads, especially in the spring.[362]

PLANTAGO MAJOR IN EUROPEAN HERBALISM IN THE EARLY TWENTI-ETH CENTURY: In early twentieth-century Britain, plaintain was applied to intermittent fevers (a remedy that has since fallen out of use).[363]

Germans of the late nineteenth century applied plantain leaves directly on wounds. And similar to the Irish, in the Tyrolean Alps folk healers soaked the seeds from the broad-leaved plant in milk as a healing drink for children suffering from dysentery.

The Czechs of the early twentieth century valued the plant's dense cluster of roots, which they prepared as a remedy against fever.

Along the Istrian peninsula during that period, Croatian and Italian folk healers cooled heat rashes by placing the plant's fresh leaves directly on the affected skin.[364]

In Romania plantain was used in spring salads during the Lenten season. Lithuanians made a wine with the juice of leaves as a medication for internal bleeding.[365]

In folk medicine in Russia and Ukraine, plantain was a remedy for bruises, cuts, and abscesses, for skin inflamations and insect bites, and as an expectorant and hemostatic agent. Fresh plantain leaves were applied to wounds, boils, cuts, and ulcers, in some cases crushed and in others applied whole to the sore spot and dressed. Alcohol tinctures of the leaves washed wounds and ameliorated toothache from cavities. Powder from plantain seeds relieved chronic diarrhea, intestinal catarrh, and even dysentery.[366]

In official Russian medicine, preparations from plantain leaves were recommended for gastritis and enterocolitis. *P. psyllium* seeds were used for spastic and atonic constipation and as a mucilage for chronic colitis. The fresh juice from the leaves was also administered in combination with sulfonamides and antibiotics for chronic colitis and dysentery.[367]

PLANTAGO MAJOR IN ASHKENAZI HERBALISM IN THE PALE IN THE EARLY TWENTIETH CENTURY:[368] *Plantago major* was a common weed found growing in meadows and glades, on heaps of refuse, and along the roadways of the Pale of Settlement. It could be found almost everywhere people lived or worked or traveled, and it was well-known and valued by the traditional medicine practitioners of Ashkenazi towns and villages for the treatment of wounds and abscesses.

In the Podolia region of present-day Ukraine, *Plantago major* was used by folk healers for boils, wounds, bee stings, and other skin-related sores.[369]

Folk healers in Polona, Ritzev, Olt-Kosntin, Cherkoss, Broslev, Ladizhin, Chopovitch, Ananiev, Balte, and Zvenigorodka could be found applying fresh or steamed dried plantago leaves directly to fresh and festering wounds, abscesses, and boils or washing a decoction of the leaves on similar injuries.

In Slovita, a tincture of the plantain's root was given by a folk healer as a mouthwash to calm toothaches.

An infusion of the whole plant including the root was a remedy for bloody diarrhea in Polona. In Kharkov occasionally only the roots and seeds or the seeds alone were used to make a tea to treat the same illness.

In Cherkoss the roots, steeped in vodka for nine days, made a trusted tincture for tuberculosis.

A decoction of the entire plant including the root was used by several folk healers for a variety of illnesses: for tuberculosis in Korosten, for shortness of breath in Polona, for heart palpitations in Bohslov, for (unspecified) heart ailments in Monasterishtche, and in Zvenigorodka for malaria.

Women were given a plant infusion to stop hemorrhage, or menstruation, in Barditchev and to help with postnatal pains and complications in Makhnivke. This styptic quality of plantain sought in Barditchev had a precedent not only in the ancients' assessment of the plant but possibly also in a medieval Hebrew remedy book that allegedly included the statement "I have heard that the juice of the plant called *wagruch*, and in French, *plantain*, is equally good when there is no olive oil," in preparing an ointment to stop the flow of blood.[370]

In Baturin the main stalk, along with the inflorescence, was brewed like tea as a gargle for colds.

A folk healer in Bohslov would make an infusion of *Plantago major* and *Verbascum phlomoides* (orange mullein) to be given as a remedy for grippe, an old-fashioned term for influenza.

Fresh plantain leaves were applied locally to erysipelas-stricken parts of the body by a healer in Zvenigorodka. This remedy recalls an ancient Greek usage of the plant.

Fresh or dried leaves covered with sour cream were a cooling plaster for wounds used by a healer in Maryupol.

The fresh leaves, ground and mixed with fresh sour cream or grease, were applied to abscesses in both Letichev and Korosten.

In Ladizhin, as if summoning the knowledge of both Hildegard and Shakespeare, a folk healer, possibly a midwife, prepared a decoction of the plant that was given to children who had sustained bone fractures.

18
POLYGONUM AVICULARE

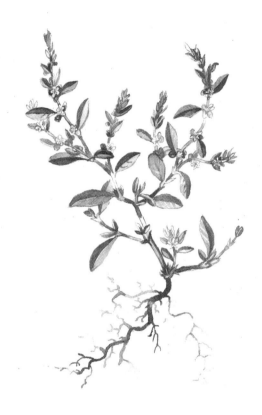

FAMILY: Polygonaceae

COMMON ENGLISH NAMES: knotweed, knotgrass, door-weed, prostrate knotweed, birdweed, pigweed, lowgrass, beggarweed, bird knotgrass, cow grass, crawlgrass, ninety-knot, ninejoints, smartweed, water pepper

YIDDISH: גריקע

HEBREW: רבברך

UKRAINIAN: Спориш звичайний, спориш, шпориш, пориш, подорожник

GERMAN: Vogelknöterich

POLISH: Rdest ptasi, rdest różnolistny

RUSSIAN: Горец птичий, птичья гречиха, спориш

LITHUANIAN: Takažolė

DESCRIPTION AND LOCATION: Annual common in waste places and cultivated soils the world over. Alternate lance-shaped leaves grow directly from swollen joints on a creeping smooth stem. Leaves are narrow at the base, which is covered by brownish sheath-like stipules or outgrowths. Scentless flowers that grow all along the stem are green and white or green with pink or purple edges and bloom from June to October. The stems easily snap at their many joints when gathered, hence the nicknames nine joints and ninety-knot.[371]

POLYGONUM AVICULARE **EARLY REMEDIES:** The earliest mentions of knotweed are from the ancients who knew this plant by many names and remedies. Its specific name, *aviculare*, comes from the Latin *aviculus* or *avis*, "bird," because great numbers of birds were known to feed on its seeds. Other later names are more humorous, like "armstrong," so called because of the difficulty encountered when one tries to wrest the plant from its habitat.[372]

In ancient Greece knotweed's astringent and cooling properties were used to stop the spitting up of blood, to treat diarrhea and cholera, and for flushing out urine for the condition of strangury. Those bitten by wild animals and those with intermittent fevers, earaches, or genital sores benefited from drinking a preparation made from the plant. For leucorrhea it was dispensed in a pessary drop by drop, and for earaches it was boiled in wine and taken with honey. As a poultice, the leaves were plastered on for heartburn, spitting blood, erysipelas, inflammations and swellings, and fresh wounds.[373]

Many centuries later the British physician William Salmon reiterated much of Dioscorides's remarks and added that "the Balsam strengthens joints, comforts the nerves and tendons, and is prevalent against the gout."[374]

Old Russian herbals of the seventeenth century mention the knotgrass as a styptic for women's hemorrhages and hemoptysis (the coughing up of blood or blood-stained mucus from the bronchi, larynx, trachea, or lungs that can occur with lung cancer, infections such as tuberculosis, bronchitis, or pneumonia, and certain cardiovascular conditions).[375]

Paracelsus described knotweed as a rubefacient, while sixteenth-century Italian botanist Pietro Mattioli documented its fresh juice as a treatment for open sores on animals to disperse flies from wounds. He also noted that putting the plant on fresh meat protected it from insects.[376]

After this era, further documentation on the plant becomes rare, and it is not until the twentieth century that herbalists begin to mention knotweed's medicinal qualities again.[377] (An interesting aside: archeological sites in Gdańsk, Poland, reveal that in the twelfth and thirteenth centuries, people living there were using *Polygonum aviculare* for dyeing both their fabrics and thread blue.[378])

POLYGONUM AVICULARE **CONTEMPORARY ACTIONS:** astringent, diuretic, hemostatic, vulnerary, anti-inflammatory, diaphoretic, rubefacient

POLYGONUM AVICULARE **CONTEMPORARY MEDICINAL PARTS:** whole plant when in flower

POLYGONUM AVICULARE **IN CONTEMPORARY HERBALISM:** In the twentieth-century United States, the plant has been recommended in decoction, infusion, or tincture form as a treatment for diarrhea, dysentery, and enteritis, as well as bronchitis, jaundice, and lung support. It has also been a remedy to stop all forms of internal bleeding, including stomach ulcers. For infants suffering from cholera with diarrhea and vomiting, the plant's use has been reported as successful. In addition, if taken consistently, the tea or tincture is reported to dissolve gravel and stones.[379] Combined with St. John's wort, knotweed is noted as controlling vomiting and the spitting up of blood.[380]

Native people of North America adopted it to treat urinary gravel, painful urination, bloody urine, and stomach pain. They also applied it topically as a poultice for pain, cuts, and inflammation. Choctaw women drank a preparation of the plant to prevent abortion, and the Chinese are also known to use this plant in their traditional medicine for pain in urination, itching, and worms.[381]

In German herbal medicine, knotweed has been included in a cough tea recipe.[382]

In the first decades of the twentieth century, a Soviet pharmacist observed how traditional healers were using knotweed preparations to stop uterine and hemorrhoidal bleeding. His research was responsible for the reintroduction of the plant into contemporary official Russian medicine. One such product, a commercial preparation available with a physician's prescription, has been used to stop uterine bleeding. For treating hemorrhoids, the plant is a primary component in yet another commercial product.

To treat headaches, Russian traditional healers harness the plant's rubefacient qualities to stimulate blood circulation to the skin by applying a compress of the fresh crushed herb to the back of the head. Taken as a tea, knotweed is a remedy for hemorrhoids and part of more complex herbal formulations for stopping internal bleeding. To reduce the swelling of hemorrhoids, a sitz bath made with an infusion of the plant can be taken. For oral support such as toothache relief or laryngitis treatments, folk healers offer an infusion of knotweed gargle. The plant's fresh juice is applied to sores and wounds to draw out infection. Moreover, the plant is valued in the care of livestock to treat open sores and rid them of flies and other insects. Herbalists, however, caution that knotweed's application should only be under the supervision of a physician or trained herbalist.[383]

POLYGONUM AVICULARE IN EUROPEAN HERBALISM IN THE EARLY TWENTIETH CENTURY: In the British Isles the plant was known to have astringent properties, and infusions of knotweed were found to be useful in diarrhea, bleeding hemorrhoids, and all hemorrhages. In addition its diuretic qualities were employed as a treatment for strangury and to expel stones. A knotweed decoction was also administered to kill intestinal worms. As a styptic, to staunch a nosebleed, the fresh juice from the plant was found to be effective when the stricken nostril was sprayed with the solution while simultaneously applying it to the temples. As a topical vulnerary ointment, the herb provided a beneficial remedy for sores.[384]

Toward the end of the nineteenth century the so-called Homero-Tea made with *Polygonum aviculare* was in great fashion in Germany and Austria and was praised as a remedy for asthma, tuberculosis, and bronchitis. Its inventor,

Paul Homero, patented his formula in 1885 as a sort of proprietary combination of *Polygonum aviculare* and *Lepidium ruderale* (or narrow-leaf pepperwort, roadside pepperweed, or peppergrass—and an herb included earlier in "Materia Medica," see p. 151), stating it was "to be used as a medicinal tea against all complaints of the throat and lungs."[385]

In Czechoslovakia a decoction of the whole plant was used in the treatment of lung catarrhs, while in Austria it was an officially government-recognized medicinal herb.[386]

In Russian folk medicine the plant was used for malaria, tumors, tuberculosis, and other diseases; it was also used as an astringent and diuretic, while the dried herb was part of an anti-diabetes tea blend.[387]

Knotweed was widely used in Ukrainian folk medicine against diseases of the kidney and liver, gastric and bladder catarrh, and diarrhea, and to treat wounds both fresh and old. It was also a key ingredient for gallstones and other "stone" diseases. According to a prominent Ukrainian herbalist: "Based on folk practice and personal observation, I have come to the conclusion that, like St. John's wort, knotweed occupies a large place in the folk treatment of most metabolic disorders of the body and a number of other diseases."[388]

POLYGONUM AVICULARE IN ASHKENAZI HERBALISM IN THE PALE IN THE EARLY TWENTIETH CENTURY:[389] In the Pale of Settlement at the turn of the twentieth century, knotweed was common along highways, near inhabited places, on rubbish heaps, and in fields—in other words, like other weeds, it grew where people lived.

In Balte, Vinitza, and Korsn, a decoction of knotweed was given by folk healers to lessen heavy bleeding, and in gynecological health midwives gave it to women suffering from heavy menstruation.

A tea made of the plant was given to people suffering from tuberculosis in Monasterishtche.

In the small towns and villages of the Pale, the plant was also well-known by traditional healers for its digestive support characteristics. A decoction of dried or fresh plant or an infusion of the plant or of the dried roots was given to children and adults suffering from diarrhea, bloody diarrhea, and stomachache in Shepetovka, Cherkoss, and Balte. In Barditchev it was given to stimulate digestion.

It is interesting to note that in Berdyansk and Mangush, two Ukrainian towns that did not have large Jewish populations, a decoction of the upper, or aerial, parts of the plant was a remedy given to those suffering from hemorrhoids and hemorrhoidal hemorrhage as a steam bath. Both of these treatments are somewhat similar to those used in contemporary Russian folk medicine.

A decoction of the plant, including the root, was used as a mouthwash to soothe toothache in Kresilev, again echoing Russian usage of the herb.

The plant decoction was drunk for kidney diseases in Anapol and as a diuretic in Berdyansk.

For lung support, in Zhitomir, Berdyansk, and Mangush the same decoction, made with the plant's aerial parts, was drunk for shortness of breath, very reminiscent of the well-known Homero-Tea remedy popular in Germany and Austria at the end of the nineteenth century.

A root decoction was a remedy for fever in Cherkoss, Savran, and Balte, much as Dioscorides recommended for intermittent fevers.

A hot, weak decoction of the flowering plant was drunk and also used in bath treatments for head colds and coughs in Zvenigorodka, Broslev, and Berdyansk; in Berdyansk this same weak tea was also given for a stomachache.

A decoction of the whole plant, including the root, served as a remedy for venereal diseases, including syphilis, in Ulan. This remedy is a distant echo of one used by the ancients and cited earlier.

A decoction was used to wash festering wounds in Cherkoss.

In Ladizhin the fresh crushed plant, occasionally mixed with *Malva pusilla* (low mallow, small mallow, or the round-leaved mallow), combined with grease was applied locally to abscesses, also somewhat similar to what Dioscorides documented some two millennia prior.

A powder of the dried plant was sprinkled on the tongue of infants suffering from thrush in Broslev, while in Olt-Kosntin a local midwife recommended that children be bathed in a knotweed decoction to ease nettle rash.

Another interesting aside is the story of Mrs. Słupowska, an elderly "Jewish woman with a Polish-sounding name," from Apt, Poland (present-day Opatów, Poland), who suffered from asthma. To treat her condition, she was often seen taking a green powder from a little wooden box. This she placed on a small dish, lit with a match, and bent over to inhale the fumes through her cupped hands.[390] It is possible the powder could have included knotweed or any number of herbs in the Pale known to treat asthma.

19
POTENTILLA ANSERINA

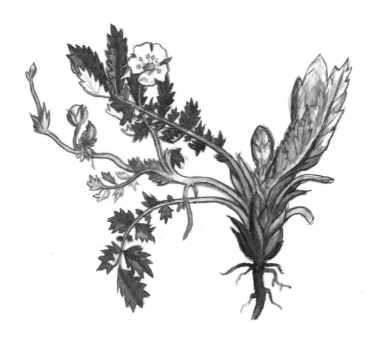

NOTE: The literature covering *Potentilla anserina* is confusing. At times some sources refer to *P. anserina* as cinquefoil. In these cases the name cinquefoil will be used. Where *P. anserina* is called silverweed in the sources consulted, it will be referred to as silverweed.

FAMILY: Rosaceae

COMMON ENGLISH NAMES: prince's feathers, silverweed, cramp weed, goose grass, wild tansy, goosewort, silvery cinquefoil, goose tansy, goose grey, moor grass, wild agrimony, five-finger blossom, sunkfield, synkefoyle

YIDDISH: פֿינגערבלאַט, געזונגבלימל

HEBREW: פּינטאַפּילון

UKRAINIAN: Гусячі лапки, перстач, гусяча лапка, гусині лапки, гусятник, біле зілля, спинки, крівавник, земляна грабинка, бедренець, чистець, перевійка, золотник, братські пальчики, вразник

GERMAN: Gänsefingerkraut

POLISH: Pięciornik gęsi

RUSSIAN: Лапчатка гусиная, гусиная лапка

LITHUANIAN: Žąsinė sidabražolė

DESCRIPTION AND LOCATION: Various species of the perennial *Potentilla* can be found in dry fields, meadows, pastures, and marshy places in both ·Europe and North America, but it is also at home throughout the temperate regions of the world "from Lapland to the Azores" and in places as far-flung as "Armenia, China, New Zealand and Chile." Roots are thin with rooting runners, and from them grow a basal rosette of compound leaves with many oblong leaflets arranged on either side of the central stem in staggered pairs opposite each other. These sawtooth-edged leaflets are green above, with silky white hairs on the underside. The hairs are also found on the plant's stem and runners, giving the plant a silvery appearance from which it takes its name. Single bright-yellow flowers bloom on long stalks from May to September.[391]

***POTENTILLA ANSERINA* EARLY REMEDIES:** The ancient Greeks understood *Pentapetes*—as their species of cinquefoil (*Potentilla reptans L.*) was known in that language for its five leaflets—to be a remedy for many illnesses including toothache, "putrid humors in the mouth," hoarseness, diarrhea, dysentery, rheumatism or "joint and hip ailments," shingles, scrofulous swellings in the glands, indurations (localized hardening of soft tissue of the body), swellings, aneurysms, abscesses, erysipelas, calluses, mange, liver and lung disease, epilepsy, jaundice, fistulas, cataracts, intestinal hernias, and excessive bleeding. The Greeks also employed this herb for atonement rituals, religious services, and purifications.[392]

In former times *Potentilla anserina* was also called *argentina*, from the Latin *argent*, "silver," because of the plant's characteristic frosted-silver appearance. Its species name, *anserina* (Latin *anser* translates to "goose"), probably refers to the fondness that geese have for the herb.[393]

The generic name, *Potentilla*, is derived from the Latin adjective *potens*, "powerful," in deference to the medicinal properties of some of the species.[394]

Hildegard wrote in the twelfth century that silverweed, or *"grensing unkrut,"* was "a weed and not of any benefit to a person's health. Thus if a person eats it, it neither benefits them nor harms them."[395]

Not long after, Maimonides, like Dioscorides, wrote only of cinquefoil (*P. reptans*), and not silverweed, which he identified as the plant known in Arabic as *nabtabilun*, after the Greek *pentaphyllon*. He also noted the rhizome and leaves were sometimes sought for their astringent qualities. Cinquefoil was still being sold in Cairo's bazaars as late as 1890.[396]

Nicholas Culpeper, whose *Complete Herbal* was published in 1653, wrote only of cinquefoil (*P. reptans*) but made no mention of silverweed (*P. anserina*). Cinquefoil is mentioned in his text twenty-seven times and described as "an especial herb used in all inflammations and fevers, whether infectious or pestilential or, among other herbs, to cool and temper the blood and humours in the body; as also for all lotions, gargles and infections; for sore mouths, ulcers, cancers, fistulas and other foul or running sores."[397]

Some decades later, Tobias ha-Kohen mentioned *Potentilla* as curing mouth and throat lesions, stopping diarrhea, easing menstrual cramps, soothing kidney complaints, and healing skin lesions, including those on the eyelids.[398] However, it is difficult to determine which species ha-Kohen refers to.

The eighteenth-century Bavarian priest Sebastian Kneipp, one of the forefathers of the naturopathic medicine movement, recommended silverweed (*P. anserina*) cooked in milk as a treatment for seizures.[399] He also observed the successful effect of the plant on menstruation, asthma, heart trouble, angina pectoris, and stomach and intestinal cramps.[400]

In the medieval Kraków region, the herb was "useful for wounds, fever, and stones." Similar to the Russian, one Polish common name for silverweed (*P. anserina*) also suggests the fondness geese have for the herb.[401]

While it's not known today as a culinary herb, early Russians ate the fresh leaves in salads and soups and considered the plant, mashed to a pulp, as a flavorful addition to various meat dishes.[402]

POTENTILLA ANSERINA CONTEMPORARY ACTIONS: antispasmodic, astringent,[403] anodyne, diuretic, emmenagogue, hemostatic, laxative, vulnerary[404]

POTENTILLA CONTEMPORARY MEDICINAL PARTS: whole plant, gathered in late spring to early summer, and dried

POTENTILLA ANSERINA IN CONTEMPORARY HERBALISM: In the West this herb's popularity has waned a bit. As late as the 1970s, one American herbalist wrote of a plant identified as *Potentilla anserina* with a common name of cinquefoil that could be boiled in either water or milk as an excellent remedy for diarrhea, and even dysentery. Cramps could also be quelled by its antispasmodic properties, especially when combined in a tea with lemon balm leaves (*Melissa officinalis*) and German chamomile flowers (*Matricaria chamomilla*). As a topical the same tea was recommended to astringe skin irritations and sore mouths and throats.[405]

In the late 1990s herbalist David Hoffmann extolled silverweed's (*P. anserina*) virtues as "an effective anti-catarrhal herb" that could be taken to decrease an overproduction of mucus. He also wrote of its well-known astringent properties for which it could be taken either internally or topically for hemorrhoids. Diarrhea when accompanied by indigestion was also an indication for this herb. Its toning and tightening properties have also served well for oral conditions such as sore throat or gingivitis.[406]

Sticky cinquefoil, or *Potentilla glandulosa*, found mostly at low elevations throughout western North America, is part of the herbal tradition of the Okanagan and Thompson tribes and understood to be a mild stimulant and tonic for rejuvenating energy. The herb has also been known to treat colic, stomach acidity, and headaches. The Gosiute people make a poultice of the leaves to treat swellings.[407]

Other related species are used by Native peoples of North America for treating ailments such as aches and pains, diarrhea, gonorrhea, mild inflammations in the mouth and throat, and excessive menstrual bleeding, and for cleaning and healing sores.[408]

Early twenty-first-century British studies showed that silverweed (*P. anserina*) continued to be used as a medicinal herb. In the Bristol area a young woman was found to be applying the herb cosmetically to wash the skin of blemishes. In Leicestershire another practitioner was found to be removing marks left by smallpox with the herb. This topical application was first recorded in the region in the sixteenth century and was again noted there at the start of the nineteenth century.[409]

Another time-honored practice in England is to wear the leaves in one's shoes to give relief from being on one's feet for extended periods of time. On the Shetland Islands the plant is only given for digestive complaints. And in parts of Ireland it is known to staunch diarrhea, help bleeding hemorrhoids and heart trouble, and "for a man's health."[410]

The contemporary Russian herbalists' name for the plant refers to its shape as resembling "goose feet." In official state medicine, it is a much-sought remedy for a varied list of ailments including spasms of the smooth muscles of the gastrointestinal tract, catarrh of the stomach and intestines, stomach ulcers, constipation, diarrhea, and dysentery.

Today folk practitioners in Russia make an infusion with the above-ground parts of the plant with goat milk for its diuretic properties, which help with kidney, bladder, and liver complaints, as well as regulate metabolism for diabetics, those with goiter, or the obese. For women who suffer from menstrual cramps, a water infusion can be helpful. As an astringent in oral health, the same type of preparation of the plant relieves toothache, bleeding gums, and sore areas of the mouth and throat. Topically an infusion made from the plant is washed on irritated skin. A decoction of the plant is also known to treat stomach problems, uterine hemorrhage, and excessive menstrual flow, as well as nervous cramps in children. In a unique preparation the dried and powdered plant is fried with eggs to treat dysentery. The juice of the plant is also taken internally for chronic inflammation of the gallbladder or can be applied topically for healing wounds, hemorrhoids, or eczema.[411]

POTENTILLA ANSERINA **IN EUROPEAN HERBALISM IN THE EARLY TWENTIETH CENTURY:** By the nineteen thirties in the British Isles, for the treatment of bleeding hemorrhoids a strong infusion of silverweed was used both topically and internally. And when sweetened with honey, it proved a beneficial gargle for sore throats. The infused plant was also a well-regarded treatment for stomach, heart, and abdominal cramps and could be either taken as a drink or applied in a compress. In Europe silverweed was boiled in milk or water to treat tetanus. A powder made from the dried leaves successfully treated intermittent fevers such as those seen in malaria. In addition the plant was beneficial as a diuretic for treating gravel, and one source wrote of it as a specific for jaundice. As an astringent decoction, silverweed also was a remedy for oral health, and a distillation of the herb was beneficial in many cosmetic skin conditions.[412]

Slovenes at the turn of the twentieth century used the plant as a plaster on wounds or even on dislocated limbs. Cinquefoil was also added into the washing basin to imbue laundry with its scent.

In Austria "five-finger cabbage" was buried under the threshold of the stable to protect cattle against hexes.[413]

Germans used silverweed as a remedy for catarrhs of the digestive tract, diarrhea, dysentery, and jaundice. Tests carried out on animals there revealed the plant possessed antispasmodic properties that affected the gastrointestinal system as well as the uterus.[414]

In Russian folk medicine the plant was used in the form of a decoction as a good astringent and fixative for diarrhea. It was also used against scurvy.[415]

POTENTILLA ANSERINA **IN ASHKENAZI HERBALISM IN THE PALE IN THE EARLY TWENTIETH CENTURY:**[416] Ashkenazim in the Pale could encounter the silverweed (*P. anserina*) in moist sandy meadows and along river banks. The above-ground parts of the plant, gathered in summer for medicinal purposes, contain a large amount of tannins and are said to have a bitter-salty and slightly tart flavor.

In folk medicine a whole-plant decoction was employed in the treatment of fever in Vinitza and Shvartz-Timeh.

In Korosten, the decoction relieved stomach ailments, diarrhea, and bloody diarrhea.

In Anapol, a midwife bathed infants suffering from indigestion in a decoction of the whole plant.

A decoction prepared from a combination of silverweed (*P. anserina*), Dnieper clover (*Trifolium borystenicum*, whose properties are similar to red clover), and meadow crane's-bill (*Geranium pratense*) was a folk healer's remedy in Anapol for stomach ailments that caused an elevated temperature.

In Cherkoss a plant decoction treated chest diseases and tuberculosis.

The same decoction was given as a sedative in Litin. In Makhnivke the same remedy was used both internally and externally for epilepsy, which echoes the plant's uses in ancient Greece.

A decoction made from erect clematis (*Clematis recta*), silverweed (*P. anserina*), and comfrey (*Symphytum officinale*) plus the leaves of guelder rose (*Viburnum opulus*) was given by a folk practitioner in the form of a steam bath for contusions and rheumatic pains. The same formula was employed as a respiratory steam for headache relief in Zvenigorodka.

A decoction of the plant was washed over affected areas to cure rash and pimples in Makhnivke, an exact replica of the folk remedy used in contemporary Bristol, England.

For sores caused by venereal diseases, a similar decoction was given in Cherkoss.

In the Pale the plant was widely used in the treatment of gynecological diseases. This mirrors a similar treatment in contemporary Russian folk medicine. Midwives made a decoction of the whole plant that was to be drunk by women experiencing menstrual cramps, and in Ritzev the plant, steamed, was applied to the abdomen of women in labor.

A plant decoction was given to drink in case of complications after delivery, and for the same purpose a steam treatment, administered by pouring the decoction over a hot stone, was known in Bohslov.

A decoction made of silverweed (*P. anserina*) and meadow fleabane (*Inula britannica*) was given to women suffering from (unspecified) gynecological diseases in the town of Zhitomir.

Children who suffered from scrofula were bathed in a plant decoction, while children and adults suffering from metabolic diseases were made to drink a similar decoction in Ulanov, somewhat similar to practices in contemporary Russian folk medicine.

In folk veterinary medicine, the boiled plant was fed to cows in Zhitomir to increase lactation.

20

QUERCUS ROBUR

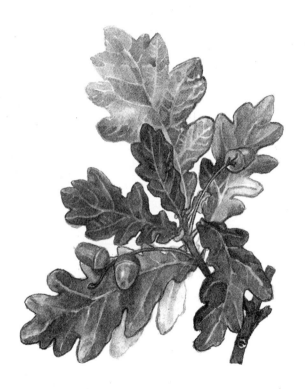

FAMILY: Fagaceae

COMMON ENGLISH NAMES: common oak, pedunculate oak, European oak, English oak, tanner's bark

YIDDISH: דעמב ,דאָמב

HEBREW: קוירקו ,קוירקוס ,קוירצי׳א ,אלון

UKRAINIAN: Дуб звичаийний

GERMAN: Eiche

POLISH: Dąb szypułkowy

RUSSIAN: Дуб обыкновенный

LITHUANIAN: Paprastasis ąžuolas, ąžuolas, ūžuolas

DESCRIPTION AND LOCATION: The European species of oak reaches heights of 115 feet. Its leaves are lobed and rounded.[417] The tree produces two types of flowers, one of which bears the fruit, or acorn, which is generally one half to one inch long. The long-lived oak is noted for both its slow growth and expansive girth; one remarkable specimen is known to have reached thirty-six feet in diameter. The famed Round Table of King Arthur was hewn from a single slice of oak, cut from an enormous bole, or trunk. In the 1930s when Maude Grieve wrote on Quercus, before contemporary testing was available, what was then thought to be the original Round Table is now believed to be a thirteenth-century replica.

***QUERCUS ROBUR* EARLY REMEDIES:** Reverence for this majestic tree reaches back to before recorded history. From the earliest documentation, we know the Greeks held the oak sacred, the Romans dedicated it to Jupiter, and the Druids venerated it. The genus name for the tree comes from the Celtic *quer*, which means "fine," and *cuez*, for "tree."[418]

The Hebrew Bible is also a source for the *Quercus* in human history, as there were at least two dozen species of oak in the region known as the Holy Land. The Hebrew words used to identify oaks were many, including *êl, elon, i'a, alah, allon,* and *elah* or *alahim*.[419] And it is believed that Abraham received the angel of Yahweh under its branches.[420]

In the northern hemisphere, every religion and mythology claimed the mighty oak as a symbol of strength. The medieval Merlin, of sorcery fame, conjured his spells beneath its canopy, as did the Druids when performing their mystical rites. The oak was also believed to provide protection from lightning, and farmers planted the tree away from their houses as a decoy for possible strikes during thunderstorms. In addition to being considered a protector from every manner of disease in humans and other animals, oak's remedial properties were described by one biblical scholar as affording "rest to the miserable Wandering Jew."[421]

One tree, the famous Oak of Mamre—a specimen of the species *Q. coccifera*, native to the countries bordering the Mediterranean—was popularly believed to represent the spot where the original tree grew under which Abraham pitched his tent. A common superstition held that anyone who cut or maimed this oak would lose their firstborn son.[422]

Medicinally the ancient Greeks knew of the entire tree's astringent properties, but they identified the membrane between the bark and the trunk and the covering immediately under the shell of its acorn as having the strongest actions. A decoction of these was given for bowel complaints, in dysentery, and for spitting blood. In women's health a powdered preparation was added to pessaries for those suffering from fluxes (an abnormal discharge of blood or other matter from within the body).

Acorns were also considered medicinal but were known to cause headaches and flatulence when eaten. Their decoction, however, was part of an antidote for venoms. In addition, ground into a poultice, acorns soothed inflammations and sores. The leaves of all oaks were chopped finely and applied to tone and tighten swellings.[424]

The ancients also made use of the oak's gall; when ground, its astringent properties were beneficial for oral health, including toothache. When heated over coals, galls provided additional styptic properties to their healing abilities and, when decocted, were used in sitz baths to treat prolapsed uterus and discharges. Other preparations were offered in cases of dysentery and bowel complaints. In general the galls were considered appropriate whenever a medical condition necessitated contracting, drying, or staunching. Soaked in vinegar or water, the galls were also used to dye hair black.[425] Maimonides later added febrifuge to the oak's list of medicinal actions.[426]

Eighteenth-century physician Tobias ha-Kohen used many terms for the tree in his description of its medicine, among them the Hebrew *ella*, the Latin *quercus*, and the German *Eiche*. His remedies are related to the tree's febrile, digestive, and urinary system actions.[427]

A bit later the Swiss physician Tissot advised using a powdered form of the part of the gall immediately under the rind to astringe bursting, open blood vessels.[428]

An old tale concerning the oak tells how the Jews settled in Poland. In the town of Kazimierz—or in the Yiddish pronunciation, Kuzmer—under a great oak tree, fourteenth-century King Kazimierz is fabled to have entertained his Jewish mistress, Esther. Legend has it that she was instrumental in the king's decision to invite the Jews to his kingdom to promote commerce there. The oak, which is believed to be almost a thousand years old, had branches so long and heavy they had to be supported to keep from breaking. The tree was still standing by the time of the Second World War and was considered a national monument.[429] A contemporary Polish author writes that this tree is just one of many thousand-year-old oaks in the town of Kazimierz, on the Wisła River, not far from present-day Kraków.[430]

The oak was considered sacred to the Lithuanians as well. Before the fifteenth century, people put offerings under the most majestic oaks to ensure themselves and their communities of health and good harvests, and the church dedicated a remarkable number of clergy orders to the worship of the oak. This practice seems curiously similar to one seen in England, where a ceremony was performed by the clergyman under the most remarkable tree at the edge of a parish to "read passages from the Gospels and ask for blessings for the people."[431]

QUERCUS ROBUR **CONTEMPORARY ACTIONS:** astringent, tonic, antiphlogistic, disinfectant, hemostatic, stomachic, styptic, vulnerary

QUERCUS ROBUR **CONTEMPORARY MEDICINAL PARTS:** bark, acorns, gall, leaves

QUERCUS ROBUR **IN CONTEMPORARY HERBALISM:** A popular American herbal of the early 1970s describes a decoction of the oak's bark as binding; it can quell vomiting and bleeding from the mouth, and its astringent properties are beneficial for chronic diarrhea and dysentery. As an antiseptic, it has been helpful as a douche or a poultice for festering sores. The acorn has its own medicinal and edible properties, and has also been roasted as a coffee substitute.[432] The oak gall too has been prized for its healing effects; Indigenous peoples of the continent are knowledgeable of them.[433] For overexertion a tea can be taken.

In twenty-first-century American practice, clinical herbalists identify white oak bark (*Quercus alba*), and that of other oak species, as a source of powerful astringents that can help with hemorrhoids and other varicosities if taken internally; however, its strong drying properties can make it constipating and are implicated in other complications if ingested long term. Topically a decoction of the bark poses no risk and can be found to help with hemorrhoids, as a douche to staunch bleeding, or as a poultice for swelling or varicosities or other bruises; as a gargle it can clear a sore throat or astringe bleeding gums. The powdered bark can be mixed with a powdered preparation of black walnut to treat bleeding gums and loose teeth.[434]

Despite its presence throughout the British Isles, *Quercus robur*'s folk medicine is predominantly sought in Ireland. Irish preparations typically require collecting the bark in spring from branches no older than five years; regional applications include as a gargle for sore throats, as a remedy against diarrhea, and as a bath to astringe excessively perspiring feet or relieve sprained ankles. Similar preparations are used for toothache, ulcers, and neuralgia or can be deployed against pinworms. In one Irish village, decocted leaves have been a preferred treatment for ringworm. Oak remedies have also been seen in folk veterinary care for horse sores and diarrhea in cattle.[435]

While British medical herbalist Penelope Ody gave the tree a very brief mention and noted its action as a strong astringent in the early 1990s, a few years later an ethnographic study in the British Isles found a handful of folk healers there remedying rheumatism and diarrhea with a decoction of the bark.[436] Another noted regional application deviated from the norm: a gargle for sore throat made with powdered acorns as opposed to decocted bark.[437]

Russian folk healers have long prescribed spending time in oak forests to promote relaxation and healthy sleep. For relieving inflammations of the throat, including hoarseness, herbalists there recommend a gargling preparation. As a mouthwash it is considered an effective treatment for inflammation of the gums, stomatitis, gingivitis, and bleeding gums. Topically compresses of a cooled bark decoction can treat many skin disorders and help reduce frostbite. Baths made from the tree's bark are recommended by folk healers for treating symptoms of allergic dermatosis (a skin condition that does not cause inflammation). For excessive perspiration of the extremities, this bath is also given, very similar to a remedy found in Ireland. A wash of the decoction is used to treat the parasitic infestation trichomoniasis, as well as inflammation of the vagina and vaginal bleeding. For addressing intestinal problems such as diarrhea, dysentery, and chronic intestinal inflammation, as well as that of the bladder or urinary tract, a bark decoction is recommended. A commercially manufactured ointment made from oak bark is applied topically to help moisturize extremely dry skin.[438]

QUERCUS ROBUR IN EUROPEAN HERBALISM IN THE EARLY TWENTI-ETH CENTURY: As late as the nineteen thirties in the British Isles, the oak's bark was still used to tan leather. In Brittany oak apples, or galls, were compressed into cakes and used as fuel.[439]

Poles baked their bread loaves on oak leaves to keep the bottoms from burning. They used acorns to make a coffee during hard times and also as a remedy for dysentery. Those weakened and debilitated from consumption and rheumatism were advised to bathe in an infusion made from the tree's bark. Bark infusions were also given to wash wounds, and an oral rinse helped relieve toothache.[440]

The Germans of western Bohemia drank oak bark boiled with water or milk for digestive issues. To avoid diarrhea, they powdered acorns, oak leaves, and plantain seed and drank these in warm beer early in the morning, after which they would fast for several hours.[441]

In Russian and Ukrainian folk medicine, oak bark was used in a decoction with alum as an astringent for gargling the throat, stomatitis, gingivitis, loose teeth, and other inflammatory diseases of the oral cavity and throat. It was also used to treat fresh burns and sun damage to the skin and mucous membranes. In Ukrainian folk medicine, the bark of young oak branches was mostly used as a strong astringent and to strengthen blood circulation.[442]

QUERCUS ROBUR IN ASHKENAZI HERBALISM IN THE PALE IN THE EARLY TWENTIETH CENTURY:[443] *Quercus robur* was the most frequently found tree growing on the right bank of the Dnieper, where the largest percentage of Ashkenazim had settled. It grew in oak groves and in *Carpinus betulus* (hornbeam, in the birch family) forests and was relied on widely for folk medicine in the region. Its bark was also used for tanning, its wood for building, and its acorns for livestock feed. The tree's leaves, buds, and young shoots were decocted as a tea substitute. In addition the oak's flowers attracted many of the bees that produced the region's honey, which was used in mead and other healing substances.

In Balte, Ananiev, and Cherkoss a decoction of oak twigs was used as a mouthwash to relieve the pain of toothache, mirroring the Russian remedy.

A decoction of the bark of an old oak was taken for the same purpose in Kolenivka.

In Letichev fresh or dry oak and *Salix cinerea* (gray willow or pussywillow) twigs were occasionally added to this decoction.

A bark tincture or a decoction of dry bark and young twigs was a remedy for bloody diarrhea given by folk healers in Bohslov, Monasterishtche, and Letichev, an application that is seen in most traditions.

In Zhitomir a decoction of the bark of young oak and young *Pyrus communis* (common pear) was drunk for dysentery, which appears in both contemporary Russian folk medicine and ancient Greek herbal texts.

In Ladizhin, a folk healer made a decoction of oak bark, *Matricaria chamomilla* (chamomile), and *Anethum graveolens* (dill) and applied the liquid as a compress to wounds as well as to the eyes, which recalls the Polish remedy.

The juice from the leaves or a decoction of fresh leaf-galls of oak found wide application in folk medicine for the treatment of herpes in the towns of Cherkoss, Zvenigorodka, Bohslov, and Zhitomir, and warts and wounds in Mirgorod.

An infusion of dried powdered acorns was given by folk healers to be taken internally for various hemorrhages, in particular by women in Mirgorod. In Mangush women were given a decoction of dried bark for the same purpose. This remedy can be seen in both the Russian and ancient literature on folk medicine.

21
RUBUS IDAEUS

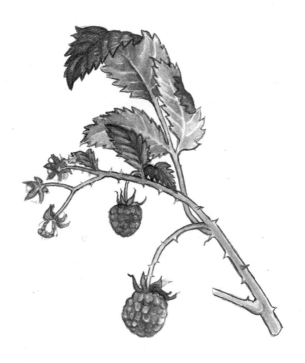

FAMILY: Rosaceae

COMMON ENGLISH NAMES: European red raspberry, garden raspberry

YIDDISH: מאַלענע, אטשענע

HEBREW: פטל

UKRAINIAN: Малина, дика малина, лісна малина, польова малина, малиник

GERMAN: Himbeere

POLISH: Malina właściwa

RUSSIAN: Малина обыкновенная

LITHUANIAN: Paprastoji avietė

DESCRIPTION AND LOCATION: Shrubby plant that can reach heights of six and a half feet, grown for its fruit but also found wild in and near forests of Europe. Biennial stems are almost thornless with compound leaves that sport three to seven toothed oblong leaflets, which are green above, often with fuzzy white undersides. In spring and summer months, the plant produces clusters of one to six white five-petaled flowers that by late summer ripen into the familiar red berry.[444]

RUBUS IDAEUS **EARLY REMEDIES:** According to Dioscorides, raspberry was given its specific name of idaeus because the plant was known to grow on Mount Ida. During his time raspberry was valued as a treatment for eye inflammations, to cool erysipelas, and as a drink with water for those with stomach problems.[445]

The noted eighteenth-century Swiss physician Samuel-Auguste Tissot, in his best-selling remedy book, included raspberry in his protocol to "cool a fever, allay thirst, correct the 'heated bile,' promote urinary secretion, and discharge and properly nourish the ill."[446]

For the most part, however, for two thousand years the raspberry lived in the medicinal shadow of the blackberry, which has traditionally been considered a vulnerary and astringent in the herbal repertoires of many cultures. It wasn't until the 1940s, when a scientific study published in the British journal *The Lancet* touted the plant's advantages if taken during pregnancy, that raspberry's healing virtues became more widely recognized.

RUBUS IDAEUS **CONTEMPORARY ACTIONS:** astringent, cardiotonic, refrigerant

RUBUS IDAEUS **CONTEMPORARY MEDICINAL PARTS:** leaves, fruit

RUBUS IDAEUS **IN CONTEMPORARY HERBALISM:** Aside from its popular status as a cultivated food, contemporary herbalists in the West value the raspberry's leaf as an astringent drunk to quell diarrhea, gargled as a mouth-wash, or washed topically for skin irritations. To treat a fever, a juice made from the fruit, sweetened with honey, is an herbal remedy. Decocted as a syrup or added to wine vinegar, this juice has also been recommended to strengthen the heart.[447]

In many parts of England and also Scotland, an infusion of the leaves is drunk at regular intervals during pregnancy to quell labor pains. British folk medicine has long held that this tea strengthens uterine muscles. Other traditional uses in the British Isles for the plant include preventing miscarriages, increasing lactation, easing menstrual cramps, preventing morning sickness, relieving both diarrhea and constipation, alleviating fevers, coughs, colds, sore throats, and arthritis, treating consumption as well as kidney stones and gravel, and washing sore eyes. In Ireland the record is less varied, with only one reported use of raspberry tea for easing a sore throat.[448]

In Germany, as in many other lands and throughout history, herbalists have found the raspberry leaf interchangeable with that of the blackberry in traditional healing, especially since the tannic acid of both plants provides the astringency needed to help with complaints of diarrhea. Extracted in hot water, the dried leaf is similar in flavor to black Indian or Chinese teas, and in lean years raspberry leaves have been fermented in the same way as Eastern teas. Some German herbalists even consider raspberry tea, which has no caffeine, healthier than black teas.[449]

In summer in Poland, marketplace stalls are piled high with red raspberries. The fruit is made into syrups, compotes, wine, preserves, liqueurs, pierogies, soups, and cake layer fillings. Much like in Germany, the dried leaves and stems have often been used to improve the flavor of other teas. An infusion of the plant's leaves is also drunk to relieve diarrhea.[450]

In Russia, where raspberry is also much loved as both food and medicine, its healing qualities are more varied.

In official Russian medicine, raspberry is considered anodyne, antibacterial, antiemetic, antiphlogistic, antipyretic, antisclerotic, appetizer, astringent, diaphoretic, diuretic, hemostatic, refrigerant, stimulant, stomachic, tonic, and vulnerary.

A tea made from the fruit treats cold and flu symptoms and acts as an antibacterial for lung inflammation. The fruit also speeds healing of gastrointestinal issues that are characterized by swelling, vomiting, pain, and bleeding. For reducing blood sugar levels in diabetes, and to treat sclerosis (abnormal hardening of body tissue), raspberries are often recommended.

Russian dermatologists recommend fresh raspberry juice or a decoction of the dried fruit, either of which can be drunk or applied topically for many skin disorders; a decoction of the leaves is used similarly.

Folk healers in Russia rely on the raspberry fruit for an even wider array of health issues, including eczema, rheumatism, anemia, diarrhea, and as a sobering tonic. For help with cold and flu symptoms, acute inflammation of the respiratory system, and erysipelas, a strong tea of the fruit and leaves is given. Decoctions of the leaf soothe coughs, tonsillitis, quinsy, and high fevers. The decocted root is also recommended for these ailments and can aid in the relief of diarrhea, asthma, and nerve inflammations as well. Combined with the flower, this preparation is advised for leucorrhea. Infusions of the plant's leaves are given by traditional healers as a vulnerary for healing acne topically or internally for inflammation of the stomach, intestines, lungs, and mouth, as well as for astringing diarrhea.[451]

In Lithuania raspberries are known to maintain the body's alkaline-acid balance and to delay atherosclerosis and hypertension. The liquid from the boiled berries is used to treat colds, promote sweating, reduce fevers, help with expectoration, and relieve rheumatism. Traditional healers there rely on the fruit to improve appetite, digestion, and the excretion of uric acid. Medicinal tea combinations can include the fruit along with other herbs such as anise and linden. The crushed leaves are also infused as a tea for upper respiratory tract ailments and gastrointestinal complaints. Gargles with the same tea help with throat and respiratory tract infections. Lithuanian herbalists caution against consuming large amounts of the plant, as too much of its purine content can cause kidney inflammation and gout.[452]

RUBUS IDAEUS IN EUROPEAN HERBALISM IN THE EARLY TWENTIETH CENTURY: In England at the turn of the twentieth century, much like Poland, Russia, and Germany, raspberries were enjoyed as liqueurs, wines, vinegars, and cooling summer drinks. And just as in those eastern lands, many in the British Isles sought raspberry infusions as remedies for feverish conditions or gargles for sore throats. A homemade wine was considered a treatment for scrofula, and the syrup, amazingly enough, was used to dissolve tartar buildup on the teeth. The raspberry's leaf was also an effective tea for oral health or for the washing of wounds and ulcerations. When combined with slippery elm bark, a poultice was applied to clean and heal both wounds and burns. And the infused leaves were a reliable drink for diarrhea or children's stomach complaints. Drunk cold, it was given for extreme laxity of the bowels. Raspberry leaf tea drunk warm was to be taken freely during childbirth as well. The ripened fruit was utilized as a fabric dye to boot.[453]

In Germany in the late nineteenth and early twentieth centuries, the fruit was given with water to those suffering from gastric disorders. Also popular in folk medicine were a syrup made from the berries, "an aromatic water," raspberry vinegar, and raspberry wine. And the thickened juice was added to improve beverages for patients.

The Slovaks placed the plant's leaves directly on open wounds as a healing vulnerary. An infusion of the leaves was also used to treat diarrhea, bleeding, and as a gargle for oral health. Saplings of the plant were used in magic medicine.[454]

In Russian folk medicine raspberry juice was deemed useful against fevers because of its acidity and tannins. Dried rasperries were also used against fever, and flowers, in the form of a tincture, served as an antidote against snake and scorpion bites. In mid-twentieth-century Russia, dried raspberries were used as a diaphoretic for colds.[455]

RUBUS IDAEUS **IN ASHKENAZI HERBALISM IN THE PALE IN THE EARLY TWENTIETH CENTURY:** I chose to include raspberry in these plant profiles because I remember it was a staple in my grandparents' house. Whenever I visited, my grandmother would always put on the table raspberry jam (with seeds included), rye bread, unsalted butter, and tea with milk. Years later my mother told me her parents would gather these fruits from the forest in the summer to sell at the weekly market in their town, Yozefov, Poland, before the war. It wasn't until I started my research that raspberries as both a food and a medicine began popping up in the most unexpected sources regarding healing in the Pale.

For example, in Vilnius, Lithuania, at Fania Lewando's vegetarian restaurant Dieto-Jarska Jadłodajnia (or Vegetarian Diet Eatery), a "fruit tea for the sick" was served. The recipe included the dried fruits of the raspberry: "Slice the peel of 1 apple and some dried apricots, and dry in the oven until brown (do not allow to burn). Add dried raspberries, and brew as a tea."[456] A raspberry syrup was also part of this restaurant's menu before it was closed during the Second World War.

In *The Shtetl Book*, which describes Ashkenazi towns in the Pale before the Second World War, under the chapter "Women's Work," a "syrup maker" is included on the short list. You can almost visualize her preparing the healing concoction with mounds of freshly gathered red raspberries.[457]

Also recalled in the same book is an Aunt Gitl, a folk healer who took care of sick children in Tishevits (present-day Tyszowce, Poland), another small town, which is about fifty miles from my grandparents' town. Aunt Gitl was beloved by her young patients because "she always prescribed the same remedy: a teaspoon of berry juice and lots of tea."[458]

And in Eishyshok, "Hayya Sorele Lubetski's daughter, Batia, for example, still swore by her mother's cure for hepatitis: a drink made of ground up raspberry vines, dandelions, carrots, followed by a drink of fresh chamomile infusion."[459]

The authors of *Life Is with People* sum up what must have been a very common occurrence: "a wealthy man, whose wife, in an effort to help her community, would supply the infirm with raspberry syrup, which was 'the marvel drug of the shtetl.'"[460]

According to another classic source on life in the Pale just prior to the Second World War, berries were a very popular commodity in Ashkenazi communities. For example, in the town of Dombrovits (present-day Dąbrowice, Poland), which is west of Warsaw and almost three hundred miles from my family's ancestral town, "an important source of livelihood for Jews were the many tons of animal pelts, the tens of thousands of pounds of mushrooms, herbs, and berries that were gathered. These products were traded both locally and for export."[461]

And finally, to underscore this plant's cultural value within the Jewish communities of the Pale, apparently counterfeit berry products were not uncommon: in Apt (present-day Opatów, Poland) there were two kinds of syrup: "the cheap one was sweetened with saccharin and artificially colored red and the good one was made with real raspberry juice and sugar."[462]

22
SEDUM ACRE

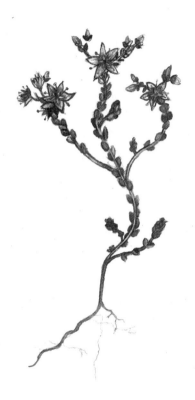

FAMILY: Crassulaceae

COMMON ENGLISH NAMES: goldmoss stonecrop, mossy stonecrop, gold moss, biting stonecrop, wallpepper, golden carpet

YIDDISH: זאַמדפֿעפֿער ,באַיסיקער ,זאַמדפֿעפֿער

HEBREW: N/A

UKRAINIAN: Очиток гострий, очиток їдкий, розхідник, ранник, жаб'ячий ліс, чистотіл, щиточки, заяча капуста, очитки-розхідник

GERMAN: Scharfe Mauerpfeffer

POLISH: Rozchodnik ostry

RUSSIAN: Очиток едкий

LITHUANIAN: Aitrusis šilokas

DESCRIPTION AND LOCATION: Perennial succulent shrub with sprawling, mat-forming stems. The plant's root is very fibrous with minute threads that are able to penetrate the narrowest crevices. Branches grow upright to eight inches with many cylindrical, short, fleshy, almost round green leaves that often overlap from crowding. Bright yellow, star-shaped, five-petaled flowers grow in clusters from leafy stems that elongate in summer. *Sedum acre* can be found cultivated in rock gardens and on walls and edgings; it also grows wild on walls, roofs, and in dry rocky places. This *Sedum* and two others were ingredients in a famous vermifuge remedy, or "theriac." The herb's name wallpepper can be attributed to its hot and peppery taste.[463]

***SEDUM ACRE* EARLY REMEDIES:** The Roman naturalist Pliny the Elder recommended that for those who sought a good night's sleep, *Sedum* should be wrapped in a black cloth and placed under the insomniac's pillow without their knowledge for the herb to have its intended soporific effect.[464]

Around the same time, the Greeks wrote of a kind of houseleek or stonecrop that grew on rocks, had a warm and sharp taste, ulcerated what it came into contact with, yet dispersed scrofulous swellings on the glands when plastered on with lard.[465]

A thousand years later Maimonides identified at least a dozen possible names from different linguistic origins for this plant and noted that its juice served in the preparation of collyria, an antiquated term for a lotion or liquid wash to cleanse the eyes.[466]

By the seventeenth century Nicolas Culpeper found wallpepper's actions to be antithetical to that of other sedums and, therefore, was opposed to any application of the herb except as a treatment for scurvy or to combat the "King's

Evil," or scrofula, while other herbalists recommended it in the form of a gargle to heal scurvy of the gums.[467]

Friedrich Wilhelm Georg Kranichfeld, an early nineteenth-century German physician and ophthalmologist, recommended the external and internal use of the plant in the treatment of catarrhs, in particular of the eye. In Germany the plant was also recommended for diphtheria.[468]

In Poland wallpepper was heated and then applied to the throat when sore. The fresh leaves were crushed to produce a poultice that was applied to cancerous sores to give pain relief; if changed frequently, it was a beneficial vulnerary. In line with Culpeper's recommendations, Polish herbalists strengthened gums affected by scurvy with a mouthwash decoction of the herb. The plant was also fried in unsalted fat to create a wound salve.[469]

SEDUM ACRE CONTEMPORARY ACTIONS: emetic, vulnerary

SEDUM ACRE CONTEMPORARY MEDICINAL PARTS: leaves, fresh or dried in warm conditions

SEDUM ACRE IN CONTEMPORARY HERBALISM: *Sedum acre* is not a plant commonly seen in contemporary Western herbalism, and documentation on its medicinal application is minimal. The handful of examples I have been able to locate have been from the British Isles. In Norfolk, England, for example, the plant was found to be used in folk medicine for dermatitis, and in Cardiganshire it has seen use in an ointment for shingles. In Ireland it was a remedy for worms and kidney troubles.[470]

English homeopathic practitioners have relied on the plant to treat hemorrhoids. The crushed leaves, fresh or in ointments, are sought as a soothing preparation for wounds, abscesses, bruises, and minor burns; however, it is cautioned that the slightly toxic internal use may cause dizziness and nausea.[471]

SEDUM ACRE IN EUROPEAN HERBALISM IN THE EARLY TWENTIETH CENTURY: Of the western sedums, the most widely used is *Sedum acre*, a European species that also grows in western North America. Because the plant will cause blistering if applied externally, or vomiting and diarrhea if taken internally, it was used only in small amounts for fever and epilepsy. Topically it was applied to lymph nodes and warts or corns to help remove them.[472]

In France wallpepper was esteemed by the common people as a vulnerary.[473]

Maude Grieve described *Sedum acre* in detail, as part of the stonecrop genus of plants, but does not give any contemporary medicinal uses of this specific herb at the time of her writing in early twentieth-century England.[474]

It is interesting to note that the plant was generally considered protective and was often grown on the roofs of houses in European countries as a charm against lightning.[475]

In Russian folk medicine, the extract from *Sedum acre* was used for heart and circulatory weakness and arteriosclerosis. The tincture was considered a remedy for epilepsy, dropsy, malaria, and fever, as well as an emetic and laxative. The fresh herb was used for external treatment of ulcers and burns. In Russian home-opathy the plant was used as a remedy for hemorrhoids.[476]

SEDUM ACRE IN ASHKENAZI HERBALISM IN THE PALE IN THE EARLY TWENTIETH CENTURY:[477] In the Soviet Union between the world wars, *Sedum acre* was not used in official medicine; but in folk medicine it was often recommended. The plant could be found in sandy and stony places throughout the Pale of the early twentieth century (note that one Yiddish name for this plant translates to "sandpepper").

In Barditchev the fruits were made into an ointment for swellings.

A dried or fresh decoction of the herb was drunk to clear up edema caused by heart ailments in the towns of Makhnivke, Birzula, and Ulanov.

Fresh or crushed, or steamed, dried, or roasted, the plant was mixed with butter and applied locally to edemas of the legs in Balte, Makhnivke, Ulanov, Zhitomir, and Kolenivka.

The fresh crushed herb, steeped in cold water or vodka, was employed as a remedy for malaria in Lochvitza, Bohslov, Cherkoss, Zvenigorodka, Kolenivka, and Ulanov.

In Slovita and Polona, the juice, raw or browned with fat, was applied as an ointment to swellings and hard abscesses.

In Zhitomir and Kolenivka, the crushed plant was applied locally to wounds.

Healing baths were made by adding a decoction of the plant and were given as a remedy for head colds in Cherkoss and in Lyubashivka. Folk healers in those towns recommended a massage with a tincture made from the plant for the same complaint.

In Bohslov the fresh plant juice was rubbed on the face to remove freckles.

23
SYMPHYTUM OFFICINALE

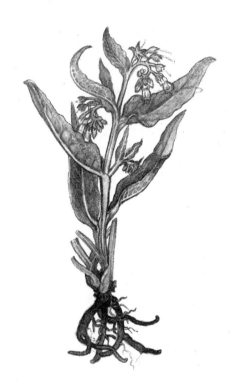

FAMILY: Boraginaceae

COMMON ENGLISH NAMES: comfrey, common comfrey, healing herb, knit-back, knitbone, salsify, consound, blackwort, bruisewort, slippery root, bone-set, gum plant, consolida, ass ear, wallwort

YIDDISH: בײנהײלער

HEBREW: קיה

UKRAINIAN: Живокість лікарський, живокість звичайний, живокість, живокіст, живокост, живокіст чоловічий, жилове зілля, стяглич, курача сліпота, живожил, болотні васильки, чорний корінь, чорне зілля, авязь

GERMAN: Beinwell

POLISH: Żywokost lekarski

RUSSIAN: Окопник лекарственный

LITHUANIAN: Vaistinė taukė

DESCRIPTION AND LOCATION: Perennial common in moist meadows and other watery places in North America and Europe. Root is black outside, white and fleshy inside, and contains a mucilaginous juice. The stem is covered with short hairs, and from it grow bristly, oblong, lance-shaped leaves, some of which are attached directly to the stem, others connected by short stalks. At the base of the plant, larger leaves lie close to or on the ground. Tube-shaped whitish or pale purple flowers resemble the finger of a glove and appear in forked, arcing clusters from May to August.[478]

SYMPHYTUM OFFICINALE EARLY REMEDIES: The very name comfrey is a corruption of con firma, a reference to a belief in the herb's ability to knit a broken bone back together. Its botanical name, Symphytum, comes from the Greek symphyo, which also means "to unite." Comfrey's healing powers have been known at least since Dioscorides's description of the herb, whose fresh root, he wrote, when taken internally, cleared up blood that was spit, and knit together flesh wounds when plastered on.[479] A thousand years later and a continent away, the German abbess Hildegard proclaimed the plant to have cold qualities and agreed that comfrey was able to quickly heal the surface of the skin; but she was not as convinced of its benefit when taken internally and cautioned against it.[480]

In the seventeenth century, British botanist, physician, and herbalist Nicholas Culpeper set down his recommendations on both internal and external applications of comfrey, finding them both beneficial, especially if the root, as opposed to the leaf, were employed. He also noted that the young leaves were commonly eaten by country people as a green vegetable or used as a flavoring agent.[481]

Paracelsus included comfrey in his alchemical observations and explained that all plants have been given their own special powers such as nutritive, bitter, cooling, or laxative. What was bestowed on comfrey, he said, is the power to heal through its consolidating quality.[482]

SYMPHYTUM OFFICINALE **CONTEMPORARY ACTIONS:** anodyne, astringent, demulcent, emollient, expectorant, hemostatic, refrigerant, vulnerary, anti-inflammatory

SYMPHYTUM OFFICINALE **CONTEMPORARY MEDICINAL PARTS:** root, rhizome, leaf

SYMPHYTUM OFFICINALE **IN CONTEMPORARY HERBALISM:** In the late 1960s and early 1970s, American herbalists were recommending the decocted rootstocks as a gargle for throat inflammations, hoarseness, or to rinse bleeding gums. As a drink it was thought to take care of excessive menstrual flow and most digestive, stomach, and intestinal complaints, or to curb the spitting up of blood. The dried and powdered root was also taken internally for blood in the urine, leucorrhea, diarrhea, gastrointestinal ulcers, dysentery, and prolonged coughs. Topically the powder acted as a styptic or in a poultice was used for the healing of wounds, bruises, sores, and insect bites. A heated topical preparation of the crushed root was applied for respiratory issues and pain caused by pulled tendons, and adding the same plant material was recommended as an ingredient in the bath "to keep skin youthful."[483] This last American recipe may have been a euphemism for the same preparation in Europe, which allegedly was a popular premarital ritual to repair the hymen and thus "restore virginity."[484]

Other American herbalists of the time identified the herb's root and leaves as being cell proliferants, capable of increasing the speed at which a wound or broken bones heal themselves. A poultice of the fresh bruised leaves was recommended to be laid on the affected area to cause the edges of the wound to knit together. In addition it was considered a remedy for asthma or rheumatism, gout, and arthritis if imbibed. A daily drink of a combination of comfrey, alfalfa, and parsley in a fruit-juice base was thought to be a tonic. For gynecological health, a douche for leucorrhea and a leaf compress for sore inflamed breasts were also considered remedies.[485]

By the early twenty-first century, laboratory studies on rats had been published showing one of comfrey's constituents had been found to be hepatotoxic, carcinogenic, and mutagenic.[486] To minimize possible risk, herbalists discouraged long-term internal use. Others remained skeptical of the studies, which were never found to be conclusive, and suggested that those interested in the herb's medicinal properties make the choice for themselves as to whether or not to ingest any preparations made from comfrey.[487] Cautions remain present in contemporary herbal publications, with further recommendations that short-term use is most likely safer than prolonged courses and ingesting the plant should be avoided altogether if pregnant, nursing, when under care for cancer or tumors, or by those with liver problems.[488] British medical herbalists also recommend this shortened-duration protocol when taking preparations of comfrey for its digestive anti-inflammatory properties.[489]

In the British Isles of the early twenty-first century, common comfrey is still a widely known folk medicine. The leaves, boiled with chickweed (*Stellaria media*), are a tonic taken for diabetes.[490] But by far the most common application of the plant has been as a remedy for sprains and strains of limbs and ligaments. In these cases the root is most often preferred, peeled, pounded or grated, and then boiled to create a thick paste that's applied as a plaster. In a less popular preparation the juice mixed with lard is rubbed onto an injury.[491]

In Germany the plant is cultivated in herb gardens. Because comfrey becomes a large and tall bush, it is thought best planted near wood strawberries, for which it has an affinity, both in the garden and in tea blends, one of which is a circulatory stimulant formula.[492]

In Poland the reputation of this herb was of such long standing that many second- and third-generation Polish Americans can recognize it as a plant grown by their mothers or grandmothers. Its most popular use was mending broken bones and for pain relief from arthritis and rheumatism. Old Polish herbals advised poulticing the leaves or washing the affected area with a decoction of the roots or leaves. In the twentieth century, folk practice included making salves by grating the root and frying it with unsalted butter until the mixture had darkened. The resulting paste was cooled and then applied to an injury. Other healers dried and powdered the root for later use such as staunching nosebleeds or preparing teas for improving digestion.[493]

At the time of the tsars, Russian soldiers used comfrey as a field remedy by mashing the roots and applying them to each other's injuries. As warfare became more sophisticated, the plant's antibacterial and styptic properties treated bullet and shrapnel wounds, and comfrey became known as the "trench herb."

Taking a cue from the West, Russian official medicine now warns against ingesting large or prolonged doses of comfrey. Official state health care uses comfrey externally for treating burns and skin grafts as well as for mending broken bones. Preparations of the plant are used to help relieve the swelling and pain of hemorrhoids as a vulnerary and styptic.

In folk medicine comfrey continues to be a trusted remedy for the speedy healing of wounds, mending broken bones, and reducing the inflammation around the site of a break. Traditional healers find the decocted herb taken internally is supportive of the digestive tract as a remedy for chronic stomach and intestine inflammation and for relieving symptoms of dysentery, gastritis, and stomach ulcers. Russian folk tradition has also known the herb to be an excellent expectorant, especially for cases of tuberculosis and chronic bronchitis.[494]

SYMPHYTUM OFFICINALE IN EUROPEAN HERBALISM IN THE EARLY TWENTIETH CENTURY: In 1912 the *British Medical Journal* recognized one of comfrey's constituents, allantoin, as having a powerful action in strengthening epithelial cells (cells that line the surfaces of the body, such as skin, blood vessels, urinary tract, or organs and serve as a barrier between the inside and outside of the body, to protect it from viruses and other pathogens), both internally and externally. At the time, the journal also reported that researchers had found a way to reproduce this substance artificially. Interestingly, nine years later another British publication, *Chemist and Druggist*, acknowledged comfrey's long-standing legacy of healing known by herbalists through the ages, yet it asserted that allantoin was a far superior medicine on its own than the entire plant had ever been. For that reason, allantoin subsequently had to be prescribed by a physician to remedy the same ailments herbalists had been healing with comfrey for at least two millennia.

In some parts of Ireland, comfrey was eaten as a cure for sluggish circulation and was regarded as a safe remedy.[495]

In France, Belgium, the Netherlands, and Hungary the root was employed in official medicine.

In official medicine in Germany, the plant was said to have a paralyzing effect on the central nervous system. In folk medicine the root was used as a decoction internally to treat bloody diarrhea and hemorrhage from the respiratory tract.[496]

In Russian and Ukrainian folk medicine, comfrey root was used for all types of inlammation of the mucuous membranes, especially for chest diseases. Comfrey root was also used as a laxative and an astringent, as well as a means of removing dead tissue and promoting tissue regeneration. It was used against colic, jaundice, goiter, and dropsy, as an appetite stimulant, and as a gargle for throat infection. It was believed that comfrey treated the kidneys and helped with diarrhea (for which a slimy root decoction was taken), even bloody diarrhea, and stomach and intestinal bleeding. It was also used for boils, ulcers, and abscesses, both internally and externally.[497]

NOTE: In Russian folk medicine, comfrey root is often referred to as *Radix consolidae* ("*zhivokost*"). It is infused in wine and drunk for various diseases.[498]

SYMPHYTUM OFFICINALE IN ASHKENAZI HERBALISM IN THE PALE IN THE EARLY TWENTIETH CENTURY:[499]

In *The Road from Letichev* comfrey is included as one of the herbs commonly used for skin disorders by healers in the Podolia region before the Second World War.[500] The Soviet field study conducted between the world wars corroborates this. In the Pale during that time, comfrey was found in moist meadows and along ditches.

In Bohslov and Polona, dry cough and lung diseases were treated by folk healers with a decoction of the root, which is close to the way Russian folk healers understood the plant.

In Chopovitch one healer would peel the young roots of the plant, cut them into small pieces, and heat them in an oven. Once they had yielded about a half glass of juice, this was mixed with honey and butter then boiled to create an elixir to remedy lung tuberculosis.

For rheumatism, colds, and contusions, a decoction of the whole plant was given as a bath and also drunk in small doses in Olt-Kosntin, Tchan, Bohslov, Barditchev, Korsn, Cherkoss, Ulanov, Zvenigorodka, Anapol, and Monasterishtche.

The root was more commonly used topically. An ointment made from the root and unsalted grease was applied locally for rheumatism, tuberculosis of the bones, and colds in Bazilia, Letichev, Kresilev, Ritzev, and Makhnivke.

A salve made from the ground fresh or boiled roots with grease was rubbed on or applied to wounds in Barditchev. The same preparation was applied locally to both humans and animals for fractures or dislocation of bones in Ritzev, Polona, Litin, Vinitza, Korosten, and Zhitomir.

In Korosten the root fried in unsalted grease was applied to bruises on the chest. These preparations are all very close to a remedy used in Poland around the same time.

A decoction of the whole plant, including the root, or of the root alone, was taken as a steam bath for contusions of the legs and arms and also to help set dislocated or fractured bones in Slavuta, Olt-Kosntin, Lachovitz, Ritzev, Monasterishtche, Broslev, Cherkoss, Bohslov, Korsn, and Zvenigorodka.

Also in Zvenigorodka, for headache complaints a root decoction was recommended to wash the head.

In Kresilev and Savran midwives relied on a decoction or tincture of the plant as a remedy for (unspecified) gynecological diseases.

24

TRIFOLIUM PRATENSE

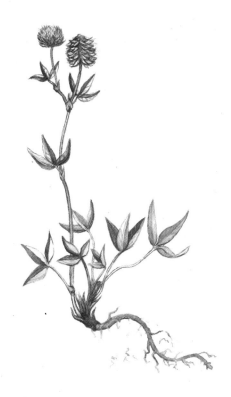

NOTE: Several species in the *Trifolium* genus were known in the Pale. The two most popular were *Trifolium pratense* (red clover) and *Trifolium repens* (white clover). Several other species are also included along with their corresponding remedies in this section.

FAMILY: Fabaceae

COMMON ENGLISH NAMES: red clover, trefoil, purple clover, wild clover

YIDDISH: קלעװער, דרײַבלאַט, קוניטשינע, קאַניטשינע, קאָנעשינע, קלאָנעשינע

HEBREW: תלתן

UKRAINIAN: Конюшина лучна, рожева конюшина, конюшинка, клевер, клевер червоний, баранчики

GERMAN: Wiesenklee, Rotklee

POLISH: Koniczyna łąkowa, koniczyna czerwona

RUSSIAN: Клевер красный

LITHUANIAN: Raudonasis dobilas

DESCRIPTION AND LOCATION: Common perennial of short duration, native to Europe, found in meadows, fields, lawns, and disturbed sites. Slightly hairy slender stems of one to two feet in height arise directly from a single root. Leaves are ternate, meaning having three leaflets, each of which is oval, almost smooth, finishing in a point and often of lighter color in the center. Fragrant flowers, from red to purple, are also oval in shape with densely packed heads and bloom from April to October. Not as popular with bees as the white clover (*Trifolium repens*).[501]

***TRIFOLIUM PRATENSE* EARLY REMEDIES:** The red clover used medicinally today was in the past mainly a fodder crop for cattle. Its familiar three-lobed leaves were associated by medieval Christians with the Trinity. The Romans used strawberry-leaved clover, *T. fragiferum,* a Mediterranean plant, which Pliny recommended taking in wine for urinary stones and prescribed the root for dropsy.[502]

Hildegard describes an unspecified clover as being as warm as it is cold and containing juice. Her general assessment of the plant as livestock fodder was commonly held, but she included one exception: as medicine for "cloudy eyes." Her remedy was to place the flowers in olive oil, stir them a bit without heating, then anoint the eyelids, freshening the mixture often and reapplying it until the condition cleared.[503] Maimonides, writing of Alexandrian trefoil, agreed with her appraisal of clover as food for beasts of burden even in Egypt around the same time period.[504]

Five hundred years later the British herbalist John Parkinson reiterated Hildegard's remedy for eye irritations but added that the plant, which could be found "in many places," yielded a "juice [that] was applied to adder bites."[505]

By the eighteenth century clover's reputation had changed again. The Padua-educated physician Tobias ha-Kohen mentions a related clover, *Melilotus albus*, or sweet white clover, in a formulation that he recommended in his section on childbirth.[506]

***TRIFOLIUM PRATENSE* CONTEMPORARY ACTIONS:** alterative, anodyne, antispasmodic, cholagogue, diaphoretic, diuretic, expectorant, hemostatic, tonic, vulnerary, nervine, sedative

***TRIFOLIUM PRATENSE* CONTEMPORARY MEDICINAL PARTS:** flower, leaves

***TRIFOLIUM PRATENSE* IN CONTEMPORARY HERBALISM:** Since the 1990s, in Britain the herb's characteristics are described as slightly sweet and cold. Medical herbalists apply the flowers mainly as a cleansing herb for skin complaints and have also found the herb useful for coughs, especially bronchitis and whooping cough, much as the Eclectics across the Atlantic had decades before. In the 1930s clover became popular as an anticancer remedy and may still be prescribed today for those suffering from breast, ovarian, and lymphatic cancers. Other folk medicine applications for red clover in the British Isles include as a fresh flower to place on bites and stings, a tincture taken for eczema and psoriasis, a compress for arthritic pains and gout, an ointment for lymphatic swellings, an eyewash with diluted tincture for conjunctivitis, a douche for vaginal itch, a syrup made from an infusion for stubborn, dry coughs, especially when mixed with other herbs,[507] a tea for nerves, and the leaves to be chewed for a toothache.[508]

Today British clinical practitioners acknowledge that *Trifolium pratense* has a wide range of medicinal characteristics, including as an application for a lymphatic and expectorant for skin and joint disease, long known in folk medicine as a "spring cleanse." Its role as part of an herbal alterative therapy in cancer management has also been recently recognized. The plant, a member of the pea family, has also had increased attention because one of its constituents has an affinity for estrogen receptors.[509] Commercial products derived from the plant have been widely promoted to help relieve symptoms of menopause such as hot flashes and also to support bone strength. Those using the plant, however, are cautioned that it contains coumarins, which may interact with prescription blood thinners such as warfarin to reduce clotting time.[510]

In the United States since the early 1970s, red clover has been planted for its nitrogen content to improve soil as a cover crop, and in herbalism it has been applied as a thick poultice to rid one of athlete's foot, in a tea for its sedative qualities, and as an alterative and antispasmodic. In addition, it's been said that to dream of a field of clover is very fortunate.[511]

American herbalists have described red clover as a diuretic and an expectorant. Tea made from the flowering tops has been recommended to stimulate liver and gallbladder activity, for constipation and sluggish appetite, or sometimes for those recovering from stomach operations to stimulate appetite. Externally, in different preparations, it has been suggested for rheumatic or gouty pains, for softening hard milk glands, and for persistent sores or other skin problems.[512]

By the last decade of the twentieth century, red clover had established its medicinal value in Western herbalism. It is considered to have a special affinity for skin conditions like eczema and psoriasis in adults and children. It is also a reliable expectorant and antispasmodic, especially in whooping cough.[513] Externally an infusion soothes burns and sores.[514]

Most recently, American clinical herbalists concur that red clover can be used in combination with other blood purifiers to address skin conditions in addition to swollen lymph glands and liver detoxification, and they concur an infusion of red clover also has a relaxing influence on spasmodic coughs. And while contemporary American herbalists agree that the plant's phytoestrogen content can possibly inhibit estrogen-dependent cancers, because of these constituents some practitioners recommend avoiding this herb during pregnancy.[515]

In Russia, after generations of only being used for dyeing fabrics, red clover has been promoted by extensive scientific research to a prominent place in official medicine as of the late twentieth century. The flowers, leaves, and root are all part of the plant's medicine. Russian folk healers use the plant to remedy anemia, emaciation, asthenia (abnormal physical weakness or lack of energy), and diabetes. An infusion of the plant encourages the onset of menstruation and soothes cramps, spasms, and uterus hemorrhage. In Russian folk dermatology a tea is drunk to address skin conditions, and externally it is known to relieve inflammation associated with the eyes or ears. In the decocted preparation of the leaves and flowers, its medicine addresses chest pain, chronic rheumatism, malaria, and kidney, bladder, and stomach issues. A traditional folk remedy decoction of the roots relieves inflammation of the ovaries and reduces benign fibroid tumors. Tincture use is associated with preventing atherosclerosis and is part of a more complex therapy for treating tuberculosis. The plant's fresh juice is drunk to remedy symptoms of jaundice and rickets. Baths augmented with the juice are given to children. It's believed that the juice from the plant, when rubbed on the roots of graying hair, restores the hair to its original color. Poulticed, the leaves can be placed on skin irritations to promote healing.[516]

In Poland the plant is known as "hair of the Blessed Virgin."[517]

TRIFOLIUM PRATENSE IN EUROPEAN HERBALISM IN THE EARLY TWENTIETH CENTURY: At the turn of the twentieth century, the American Eclectics attributed antispasmodic and expectorant properties to clover and looked to the plant for the treatment of whooping cough and bronchitis. It was also an ingredient in an ointment applied topically for ulcers.[518]

In the British Isles as well, the fluid extract of *Trifolium* was used as an alterative, and its application continued as an antispasmodic in cases of bronchitis and whooping cough. By the 1930s, fomentations and poultices of the herb had become more widely accepted as local applications to treat cancerous growths.[519]

In Russian folk medicine, preparations from red clover were used as a diuretic and expectorant, for cleansing and strengthening the blood, against colds, and in women's health, or externally as an antiseptic for wounds and ulcers. It was also used as a poultice for abscesses and burns.[520] In official medicine in the Soviet Union, red clover was used as a diuretic, expectorant, and "blood cleaner." It was known to strengthen against colds and to address female ailments. Externally it was applied as an antiseptic for wounds and skin infections.[521]

TRIFOLIUM PRATENSE IN ASHKENAZI HERBALISM IN THE PALE IN THE EARLY TWENTIETH CENTURY: *Trifolium pratense*, red clover, was one of ten clovers that were used in the folk medicine of the Pale between the world wars. Red clover was second only to *Trifolium repens*, white clover, which is addressed in the next section. Red clover was common in meadows and among shrubs of the region inhabited by the Ashkenazim. In the early years of the twentieth century, its flowers and upper leaves were gathered and dried for commercial purposes, most likely by villagers. The red clover harvests were exported in large quantities, mainly to Germany, for their production in medicines taken for respiratory disease.

In the folk medicine of the Pale, prior to the Second World War the entire plant was used.

In Cherkoss a whole-plant or flower decoction was drunk by women to induce menstruation.

The powdered dried flowers were employed by women to address (unspecified) gynecological diseases and leucorrhea in Bohslov, Polona, and Bazilia.

As a stomachache remedy a tea made from the whole plant was taken in Bohslov.[522]

TRIFOLIUM REPENS

FAMILY: Fabaceae

COMMON ENGLISH NAMES: white clover

YIDDISH: קלעװער, קאָנעששינע

HEBREW: N/A

UKRAINIAN: Конюшина біла, конюшина повзуча, біла конюшина, біла конюшинка, конюшина, клевер білий, горішки, горошок, орішина, орішина біла, білі коснички, кіснички, волошки

GERMAN: Weißklee, Kriechklee

POLISH: Koniczyna biała, koniczyna rozesłana

RUSSIAN: Клевер ползучий, клевер белый, клевер голландский, кашка белая, амория ползучая

LITHUANIAN: Baltasis dobilas

A creeping, drought-tolerant, fragrant perennial that, compared with red clover *(Trifolium pratense)*, bears larger leaves and white or pinkish flowers, not to mention is preferred by bees. White clover was common in the Pale and could be found growing in fields, dry meadows, and forests and was also cultivated in gardens.

In the West white clover has traditionally been more widely recognized for its attractiveness to bees in their production of honey than as a medicinal plant.[523] In the late twentieth century in the British Isles, a handful of folk healers were documented applying dried white clover, smoked in a pipe, as a remedy for coughs and toothache.[524]

In Russian folk medicine infusions from white clover inflorescences served as a remedy for gynecological diseases, colds, tuberculosis, and rheumatic pains. Tinctures of the flowers were also used for gynecological diseases, hernia, tuberculosis, and colds.[525]

Of the ten clover species identified in traditional healing in the region of the Pale, *Trifolium repens*, or white clover, showed the most usage in towns and villages with the highest populations of Ashkenazim. It was easily found in fields, dry meadows, and forests. Because it attracted bees, it was helpful in the production of honey, an important medicinal substance in the repertoire of all healers of the Pale. Honey was also prized in the making of mead, a popular beverage among Ashkenazim. Prior to the 1930s in the Soviet Union, white clover flowers were gathered and dried then exported for the manufacturing of remedies to treat rheumatic pain and asthma. At the time of the Soviet surveys, however, the herb was used exclusively in folk medicine.

In Kresilev and Olt-Kosntin, an infusion of the stems or flowers was given by folk healers to those with head colds and cough.

To stop heavy menstruation or postnatal hemorrhage, midwives in Korosten, Savran, Zhitomir, and Ulanov gave their patients a flower infusion or plant decoction of white clover.

In Korosten, Savran, Chopovitch, and Polona the same preparation was also given to induce menstruation.

In Cherkoss, Zhitomir, Korosten, Litin, Letichev, Bazilia, and Polona folk healers gave their patients formulations for leucorrhea.

Many other species of *Trifolium* were known remedies to folk practitioners in towns and villages of the Pale of Settlement, seven of which are listed here:

Trifolium Arvense (English: rabbitfoot clover; Ukrainian: Котики, конюшина польова, коточки)[526] was used for diarrhea in Litin and Zaslov; kidney ailments were remedied by this herb in Litin; gynecological ills including leucorrhea were helped by the herb in Polona; heavy hemorrhage was treated in Kolenivka; during delivery, if the placenta did not pass, a preparation of the plant was given in Litin; plant ash was sprinkled on rash and blackheads in Chopovitch; prepared like a tea, it was taken for colitis with resultant constipation in Kharkov.

Trifolium Medium (Engish: zig-zag clover or mammoth clover; Ukrainian: Конюшина середня, червона конюшина, червона лісова конюшина, клевер, конюшина, клевер польовий, клевер дикий, кливорот, лісова конюшина, лісна конюшина, трилистник) was used by women to stop menstruation in Balte; a strong flower and leaf decoction was given to girls to induce menstruation in Ananiev, Letichev, and Barditchev; a preparation was given in case of complications after childbirth in Khmelnik; for leucorrhea it was known to midwives in Korosten; children with scrofula were bathed in a decoction of the plant in Bazilia; a formulation of the plant was a remedy for mad dog bites in Litin and Chopovitch and given to both humans and animals.

Trifolium Alpestre (English: owl-headed clover; Ukrainian: Конюшина альпійська, конюшина альпейська, червона конюшина, конюшина, конюшинка, горішина трилистник, клевер) was formulated for consumption and cough in Vinitza; women were given a preparation to stop hemorrhage in Polona and Lachovitz; and the plant served as a remedy for leucorrhea in Korosten.

Trifolium Pannonicum (English: Hungarian clover; Ukrainian: Конюшина угорська, конюшина паннонська, біла конюшина) was prepared in a treatment for leucorrhea in Polona; children with scrofula were bathed in a decoction of this clover combined with *Trifolium medium* (zig-zag clover) in Bazilia.

Trifolium Montanum (English: mountain clover; Ukrainian: Конюшина гірська, біла конюшина, біла конюшина польова, одкасник, чортополох) was administered as a sedative after a shock in Ladizhin, oddly reminiscent of an obscure American remedy noted in the 1970s; the plant preparation was a remedy for leucorrhea in Lachovitz and Khmelnik; for paralytic symptoms after delivery, a preparation of the plant was given by midwives in Kolenivka; and it wa a remedy for dizziness in Anapol.

Trifolium Elegans (English: Alsatian clover; Ukrainian: Конюшина струнка, рожева конюшина, розова конюшина) in an infusion of stems and flowers addressed leucorrhea in Polona; a preparation made from the plant was used to induce menstruation in Letichev.

Trifolium Strepens (English: hop clover or yellow clover; Ukrainian: Хмелик польовий, конюшина шарудлива, конюшина, конюшинка, конюшник від жовтяниці, рубашишне, жовте зілля, польова крутовина, польовий клевер, тародай, дикий клевер польовий, дикий чай, польовий хмелик, дикий хміль) was used as treatment for jaundice in Korosten and Chopovitch and for cough in Barditchev; stomach ailments and nervous diseases were treated with a preparation of this clover in Khmelnik; a tea brewed of the plant with the addition of rose petals was drunk as a remedy for leucorrhea in Makhnivke, for heavy hemorrhage in Chopovitch, and for the treatment of rabies in Barditchev for humans as well as cattle.[527]

25
URTICA URENS

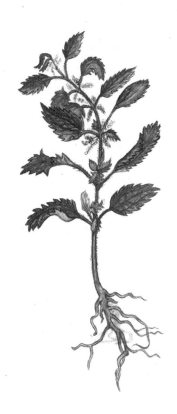

FAMILY: Urticaceae

COMMON ENGLISH NAMES: annual nettle, dwarf nettle, small nettle, dog nettle, burning nettle, stinging nettle

YIDDISH: קראָפּעװוע, קראָפּיװוע

HEBREW: אורטיקה, סרפד

UKRAINIAN: Кропива жигавка, кропива жалюча, кропива дрібненька, кропива дрібна, дрібна кропива, кропивка, кропива жалка, кропива жижавка, жижавка, гижавка, джигавка, жигалочка, жигалка

GERMAN: Brennessel

POLISH: Pokrzywa żegawka

RUSSIAN: Крапива жгучая

LITHUANIAN: Gailioji dilgėlė

DESCRIPTION AND LOCATION: Stinging nettle is a wind-pollinated perennial plant found in most temperate parts of the world, growing in woods and forests, riverbanks, field edges, disturbed areas, along roadsides, and wherever the nitrogen content of the soil is high. Its square bristly stem reaches from two to seven feet in height with opposite, pointed, deeply serrated leaves with fuzzy undersides. Tiny round greenish flowers hang from the point where the leaf attaches to the stem in drooping clusters from July to September.[528] The dwarf or small nettle, *Urtica urens*, is an annual, similar in appearance and medicinal qualities to *U. dioica*; it is also the species valued in homeopathy.[529]

URTICA URENS **EARLY REMEDIES:** It's said the Roman nettle *(Urtica pilulifera)* was introduced into Great Britain and possibly various other parts of northern Europe by Caesar's soldiers; to increase circulation and warm themselves in weather conditions they were unaccustomed to, they beat the uncovered parts of their legs with nettles. And of the four species found in the lands described in the Bible, the Roman nettle's sting is fabled to be the most irritating. As far as religious scholarship is concerned, however, there seems to be no agreement as to which word in the Hebrew Bible refers to the nettle species.[530]

    The ancient Greeks knew two types of nettle, one wilder and rougher than the other, but the leaves of both could treat dog bites, gangrene, sprains, growths, swollen glands and abscesses, spleen disease, and nosebleeds. A combination with myrrh in a pessary was employed to provoke menstruation, and the new leaves themselves were understood to have the ability to set a prolapsed uterus right. The ancients found the plant's seed to be an aphrodisiac, a respiratory aid, laxative, carminative, diuretic, and soother of an inflamed uvula.[531] And as the

Romans were aware, its calefacient properties were availed by grinding up the leaves and smearing them with olive oil or grease on affected areas of the body that needed warming up.[532]

A millennium later, German abbess Hildegard praised the herb's abilities as a cooked food to purge mucus from the stomach, as a vermifuge, and as an aid to strengthen memory. For the care of horses, she also considered the plant helpful for coughs and stomach pain.[533] Around the same time period, Maimonides documented the Arabic and Spanish names for the plant, one of which translated as "kernels of women" and another as the "plant of fire." The seeds of the small nettle (*Urtica urens*) and the Roman nettle (*Urtica pilulifera*) were both said to be sold in the bazaars of Cairo as diuretics and emollients.[534]

Slavic peoples have considered the nettle plant magical since ancient times. It protected the house against evil when hung above the entry. The herb was believed to disperse the clouds of impending storms and, when burned, warded off lightning. In the early Middle Ages even clothing made with nettles was worn to guard against demons by frightening them away.

The Polish herbalist and botanist Simon Syreniusz wrote that nettle leaves soaked in wine "cleansed the stomach, removed rumblings of the intestines and young nettle cooked with snails softened the stomach." He also recommended a nettle antidote for hemlock or animal bite poisonings. Gout, hemorrhages, colds, flu, and tired feet were treated with the herb, and it was also known to be a diuretic, alterative, hepatic, emmenagogue, astringent, nervine, and hair tonic.[535]

In seventeenth-century Russia the plant's application was mainly for treating wounds. A translation of an herbal from the era describes how nettle was chewed and applied to fresh wounds to clean and heal them. For infected conditions, the same source advised mashing both the seeds and leaves with salt to remove any dead tissue before healing could occur.[536]

Some believed that those who gathered nettles before dawn and fed them to cattle protected their livestock from evil spirits.[537]

URTICA URENS CONTEMPORARY ACTIONS: anti-allergenic, anti-inflammatory, antihistamine, diuretic, mineralizer, nutritive, tonic

URTICA URENS **CONTEMPORARY MEDICINAL PARTS:** leaves, tops, seeds, rhizomes, roots

URTICA URENS **IN CONTEMPORARY HERBALISM:** Many of the properties contemporary herbalists ascribe to nettle are similar to those described by the ancients: circulatory stimulant; amphoteric for lactation (meaning it will stimulate milk production if lacking or reduce if it's excessive in breastfeeding mothers);[538] emmenagogue; diuretic suitable for rheumatism, gout, kidney stones, and retention of urine; digestive stimulant to strengthen the stomach, intestines, liver, pancreas, and gallbladder; vermifuge; styptic to stop bleeding of all kinds; and antibacterial as a gargle for oral infections.[539] In the ancient practice of urtication, or "self-flagellation," the topical application of the leaf is still advocated by contemporary herbalists for the temporary relief of inflammation, pain, and stiffness brought on by myalgia and osteoarthritis.[540]

In the more recent past, science has discovered that the humble nettle contains many of the essential vitamins and minerals needed to maintain vitality, and most Western contemporary herbalists even consider the plant on par with TCM's "long life" herbs.[541] With these beneficial qualities, the nettle has the ability to improve a wide range of chronic health conditions that today are exacerbated by the modern diet, one too often lacking in the kinds of nutrients needed for good health.[542]

Contemporary Western herbalists not only apply the ancients' knowledge of this herb but also look to nettles for their natural immunity-enhancing properties that protect from pathogenic infection, especially when taken as a tea at the start of a feverish ailment. The plant also offers an antihistamine effect, valuable for treating hayfever and other allergies and for helping reduce the severity of asthma attacks. Nettle is helpful for regulating blood sugar levels in the treatment of diabetes and assists in lowering high blood pressure by dilating the peripheral blood vessels and promoting the elimination of urine. Because its high iron content is very easily absorbed and assimilated throughout the body, those with anemia benefit from taking nettle preparations.[543] The fresh leaf juice can be applied to skin for sores, infections, rashes, and warts. To prevent hair loss, the whole plant can be decocted and mixed with vinegar for a restorative scalp rinse.[544]

Today the plant has become a specific for treating eczema in children, especially nervous eczema.[545] It is also helpful for soothing the growing pains of young children when their bones and joints ache, similar to that of their elders.[546]

Clinical studies of nettle leaf show its efficacy when taken both orally and as a topical for relief of osteoarthritis and allergic rhinitis. Extrapolations from pharmacological studies demonstrate nettle leaf's benefit as an anti-inflammatory with broad activity including inhibition of cytokines (protein molecules released by cells that signal the immune system and inflammatory responses to become activated). Nettle leaf may also provide a source of absorbable silica.[547]

For the genitourinary system nettle is an excellent reproductive tonic for men and women, and it can be used for alleviating the symptoms of premenstrual syndrome and menopause. Studies show use of the root improves the flow of urine, reduces frequency and volume of residual urine, and, taken on its own as a tincture or with saw palmetto (*Serenoa repens*), has been successful in treating the early stages of benign prostatic hyperplasia by inhibiting cellular proliferation in affected tissue. In addition a tea made from the root can be used for hives, itch, and dysentery.[548]

Today traditional Russian folk healers work with the root to relieve cough, while the leaves have a broader application including topically as a styptic and a hair tonic; internally it is considered helpful for relief of menstrual cramps and other gynecological issues. A whole-herb decoction is given for headache relief or to support the heart, liver, and kidneys, and it's also recommended for treating gastritis and anemia. To reduce blood sugar, diabetics are given a preparation using the herb's flowers.

Contemporary herbalists in the former Soviet Union recommend infusions made with nettle for many gastrointestinal ailments including diarrhea, constipation, inflammation of the small intestine, stomachache, indigestion, and meteorism (a rapid accumulation of gas in the intestine), as well as liver, gall bladder, and urinary conditions.

In official Russian medicine, physicians have found the plant to be effective for toning the cardiovascular system, specifically for reducing cholesterol levels, treating malaria, and as part of a protocol to remedy tuberculosis. Dermatologists recommend infusions of the plant for addressing a range of skin irritations including eczema, psoriasis, and acne.[549]

Lithuanian folk healers work with nettles in much the same way as other Eastern European herbalists, seeking its spring tonic effect when the plant re-emerges after a long winter slumber. During times of war nettle was especially sought to stop blood loss from battle wounds. In more contemporary times Lithuanians have found the plant improves the production of hemoglobin and erythrocytes, reduces inflammatory processes, cures rheumatism, gout, and angina, is helpful for the prevention of stones, strengthens the gums, and treats metabolism disorders, anemia, atherosclerosis, liver and gallbladder disease, and constipation.

Folk medicine practitioners apply nettle leaves' fresh juice to cure osteomyelitis (infection of the bone), uterine and nasal bleeding, and the coughing up of blood. For diabetics, preparations of the plant are employed to lower blood sugar, and infusions of the fresh plant increase urine and clear skin conditions. For severe coughs, folk healers recommend a root decoction made with honey or sugar.[550]

URTICA URENS IN HERBALISM IN THE EARLY TWENTIETH CENTURY: Across the Atlantic, American Eclectic practitioners of the latter half of the nineteenth century and early twentieth century continued the traditions set out by the ancients and considered nettle leaf and root to be a blood purifier, styptic, stimulating tonic, and diuretic. They used the plant to treat diarrhea, dysentery, discharges, chronic diseases of the colon, and chronic skin eruptions.

In the British Isles are found two species of nettle, *U. dioica* and *U. urens*, and both have long enjoyed a contentious relationship with the humans among whom they grow. Many children were taught that the juice from the leaf of the dock plant (*Rumex crispus*), which often grows in close proximity to nettles, would give instant relief from nettle stings, and they memorized a verse to help them remember the antidote: "Nettle in, dock out. Dock rub nettle out!" It is also true that the juice of the nettle leaf provides an antidote for its own sting, as does rubbing the affected body part with rosemary, mint, or sage leaves. I have also found fresh mullein leaves to be effective.

Nettle was the subject of some intrigue during the early part of the twentieth century when Britain secretly investigated its cultivation by the Germans for both civilian and military use. By 1918 British authorities wondered whether Germany's increased interest in the herb revealed very straitened circumstances rather than any recognition of a true value in the plant for making textiles. When Maude Grieve wrote in the 1930s, she noted nettle's shortcomings in the manufacture of textiles and instead acknowledged its potential for the papermaking industry. But she concluded her lengthy entry on this plant on a more concerning note. As the plant spread across the country, causing many to demand its eradication, she described a comment in the 1926 diary of the Royal Horticultural Society that promised members "if Nettles are cut down three times in three consecutive years, they will disappear." Fortunately for contemporary herbalists, this promise seems not to have come to fruition.

British countryfolk of her time were still gathering the plant as a potherb, and Grieve's entry includes a recipe for a nettle pudding and a nettle beer. Country people were also known then to use the plant to arrest bleeding from the nose, lungs, or stomach, and many took a nettle tea as a spring tonic and blood purifier, for gouty gravel, gout, chicken pox, and bruises, and, for chronic rheumatism, practiced the age-old "urtification" techniques.

In folk medicine of the early twentieth century, nettle was a respiratory aid, both as an electuary or smoked, a remedy for tuberculosis, ague (or malaria), goiter, and obesity, a questionable diuretic, and a hair tonic. The plant was also considered a healthy dietary supplemental food for livestock, especially malnourished horses and pigs. If included in chicken feed, it increased egg production and the seeds fattened fowl. Other uses for the plant included its substitution for rennet in cheesemaking and the dyeing of fabric.[551]

In France *U. urens* was the preferred medicinal species. There, a nettle tincture was used for burns and as an extract for neglected herpes, eczema, leprosy, and psoriasis. A nettle infusion was used as a diuretic as well as a styptic.

In Czechoslovakia and Germany the nettle leaf was considered a diuretic and an astringent to remedy catarrh of the digestive tract and bladder. In Denmark ground dried seeds were added to feed for horses to maintain their health.

In Germany fresh nettles were applied to the body as a remedy for paralysis, neuralgia, rheumatism, and inducing menstruation. A seed emulsion or an infusion of flowers and plant tops was drunk for diarrhea, stomachache, and complaints concerning the neck, chest, and lungs. The plant was considered a circulatory stimulant and alterative, and the hair was strengthened by rinsing it with a solution made from the plant's roots.[552]

In Slovakia the small nettle, or *U. urens*, had its own applications: a decoction of the herb was drunk as tea against uterine bleeding; the dried plant was burned as smoke medicine to reduce swellings.[553]

In Russian folk medicine, infusions and extracts from the leaves were used as antipyretic, diuretic, antirheumatic, and antitussive agents, for anemia and dysentery, and for hemorrhoids.[554]

URTICA URENS IN ASHKENAZI HERBALISM IN THE PALE IN THE EARLY TWENTIETH CENTURY: Nettles were a common weed in the Pale, growing on rubbish heaps, along highways, in orchards, and cultivated in kitchen gardens. Folk healers considered the medicinal qualities of *Urtica urens* very close to that of *U. dioica*, and in folk medicine between the world wars, various parts of the plant as well as the whole plant were in wide use.

In Letichev, Anapol, and Kharkov, traditional healers made a drink from the pure juice of the entire plant mixed with fresh milk or a decoction of leaves and rootstocks as a remedy for cough, chest ailments, asthma, and haemoptysis.

A decoction of the plant, including the flowers, combined with its close relative *U. dioica*, was a drink for cold and cough in Lachovitz, Kresilev, Tchan, Vinitza, and Ladizhin.

Nettle stalks, leaves, and seeds were used to sting, rub on, or apply to aching parts of the body for those with colds, rheumatism, and anaemia in the communities of Romen, Uman, Polona, and Zvenigorodka. I can confirm this use after speaking with a Jewish man from Riga, Latvia, who survived the Second World War. He told me it was common for those with arthritic pain to rub themselves with nettle. This is the "urtication" method passed down from the ancients. This remedy was also given for easing spasms in Lyubashivka by the opshrekherin healer there (see afterword, p. 258).

A plant or root decoction was given as a bath for the treatment of rheumatism in both Broslev and Monasterishtche and as a foot steam bath for swellings and edema in Maryupol.

In Cherkoss whippings with steamed whisk brooms of nettles were administered and nettle juice diluted with vodka was drunk to cure fever.

In the town of Yelisavetgrod, for those suffering from a cold, the nettle's dried flowers mixed with lard were made into an ointment and rubbed on the legs after a foot steam bath (see p. 19).

In the towns of Olt-Kosntin and Khmelnik, midwives gave women who were suffering from heavy menstrual flow a decoction of the whole plant, or of the flowers only, to drink.

During the First World War, in Shepetovka, compresses of a nettle tincture were applied to the throat and rubbed on the chest and arms of poison-gas victims to give relief from coughing.[555]

26

VIOLA MIRABILIS

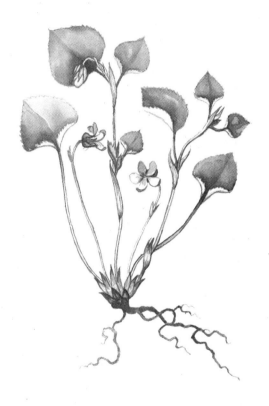

NOTE: In the Ashkenazi towns and villages of the Pale, several *Viola* species were sought for their healing properties. While *Viola odorata* is the most commonly found species in herbal sources, it was not the plant Ashkenazi healers knew. Because all *Viola* species have similar medicinal qualities, and because *V. odorata* is the best documented, the following historical comparisons will refer to *V. odorata*. *Viola* species known by Ashkenazi folk healers in the Pale can be found at the end of this section.

FAMILY: Violaceae

COMMON ENGLISH NAMES: violet, miracle violet

YIDDISH: פֿיילכל, פֿיִאַלקע, פֿיאַלקע

HEBREW: ויאולאַט, ויִאולאַיִש, סגל

UKRAINIAN: Фіялка пахуча, фіялка запашна

GERMAN: Veilchen, Duftveilchen, Märzveilchen, Wohlriechendes Veilchen

POLISH: fiołek wonny

RUSSIAN: Фиалка душистая

LITHUANIAN: Kvapioji našlaitė

DESCRIPTION AND LOCATION: (this description is mainly for *Viola odorata):* most *Viola* species are small herbaceous perennials native to Europe and grow wild in meadows, thickets, hedges, along roadsides, and at the edges of woods; they are also commonly cultivated in gardens. The plant's creeping rootstock sends out runners that also take root. Typically leaves are heart shaped and slightly downy, especially the undersides, with rounded, toothed margins, and grow in a basal rosette. The young leaves begin life rolled up into tight coils on either side of the leaf, unfurling as they mature. Bright flowers bearing five unequally sized petals can be violet, white, or rose-colored, grow on long thin stems, and include a little tail on the underside called a "nectar spur." Flowers bloom from February to May.[556]

VIOLA EARLY REMEDIES: The Greeks called the violet *Ion*, and it was said that the god Jupiter created the fragrant flowers for his love, Io, for whom they named the plant. The English term *violet* comes from *Vias*, which translates to "wayside."[557]

Pliny the Elder prescribed a liniment of violet root and vinegar for gout and disorders of the spleen, and he recommended that a garland of the flowers worn on the head would not only rid a person of the fumes of wine but also prevent headache and dizziness.[558] The ancient Greeks were pragmatic in their description of the herb and found it "to moderate anger," to bring on sleep, and "to comfort and strengthen the heart." In addition the Athenians acknowledged its cooling properties and its ability to soothe heartburn and mucus membrane inflammations, and they believed that when drunk infused in water, it could alleviate epilepsy in children.[559]

All violets have health-giving properties for a variety of ailments great and small and can be formulated many ways, and humans have long known the species' affinity for healing ailments, particularly those of the lungs, urinary tract, and skin. In North America, before written records, Native peoples worked with the plant topically to wash sore and swollen joints, received it as a tea for stomachache and asthma, and applied the flower as a poultice to relieve internal pain in the torso.[560]

In the twelfth century the abbess Hildegard made an oil with the flowers to cool inflamed eyelids and make the cloudiness "flee" from them. In addition she observed that if someone who is "oppressed through melancholy with a sad mind and is thus harmed in his or her breathing" drinks a blend of violets and wine, this medicine will make them happy and make "his or her breathing healthy."[561] Like so many of her observations, Hildegard's recognition of the correlation between the lungs, or breathing, with sadness, or a heavy heart, seems extraordinarily visionary. The pairing of the lungs with grief or sadness is a core tenet in TCM. Today many contemporary Western herbalists recognize the wisdom in this heart-lung connection and often take it into consideration when working with clients who have breathing concerns.

Nicholas Culpeper, half a millennium later, reiterated many of the ancients' findings and, like the abbess, still found violets to have cooling properties capable of soothing inflammations to ease constricted breathing. He also added the plant's ability to lessen headaches brought on by sleeplessness, its applicability in easing a hoarse throat, and its affinity for the urinary system.[562] When Tobias ha-Kohen set down his medical text, he connected violet's healing virtues with the urinary tract, including the treatment of stones, and offered a formula that mixed the herb with licorice root to cool the kidneys. He also found the plant helpful with asthma, teething, and digestion in children. Combined with poppy, plantain, and shepherd's purse in water, violet was a beneficial women's medicine.[563]

VIOLA **CONTEMPORARY ACTIONS:** diaphoretic, emetic, expectorant, laxative

VIOLA **CONTEMPORARY MEDICINAL PARTS:** flowers, leaves, roots

VIOLA **IN CONTEMPORARY HERBALISM:** In the United States, herbalists writing in the 1970s through the present day have continued to honor the legacy of the ancients with their understanding of violet as a cooling plant that helps an ailing respiratory tract, soothes inflamed mucosal tissue, calms headaches, and addresses insomnia.[564] Clinical herbalists add the species' lymphatic strengths and its demulcent qualities to the herb's repertoire of healing abilities.[565]

In England folk healers make violet flowers into a pudding that is eaten to cure "giddiness," or they concoct a syrup that is considered sedative and also mildly laxative. In some counties, records show traditional healers' use of the plant in treating cancer and ulcers and as an astringent for skin conditions, including as a counterirritant for insect stings. In Ireland the plant's application has been more restricted to tumors, as a poultice for boils, or as a decoction for the relief of headache.[566]

In Germany herbalists prescribe the herb in a recipe for Migraine Tea:

6 parts rosemary leaves

4 parts peppermint leaves

4 parts balm leaves

4 parts sweet violet

3 parts feverfew

½ part sweet violet flowers[567]

Russian herbalists use a related species, *Viola tricolor*, the wild pansy. Its nickname is "Anuta's eyes" because the flower suggests a laughing, happy face. As in the West, herbalists in Russia and Poland look to this herb to address respiratory ailments.[568] Russians also work with the plant to reduce inflammation of the urinary tract, and the herb is a common folk remedy for treating kidney stones. An infusion of the flower is a treatment for inflammations in the gastrointestinal tract and to address symptoms of dysentery. In addition Russian folk healers recommend infusions of the herb for atherosclerosis, arthritis, rheumatism, gout, rickets in children, and as a preventive for those who have suffered heart attacks. A tea sold commercially in Russia under the name Averin is to be taken internally for cough, and externally washes and compresses with the product are used to treat many skin diseases. For relieving toothache or as a wash for swellings in the mouth, dentists recommend rinsing or gargling with the same tea.[569]

VIOLA IN EUROPEAN HERBALISM IN THE EARLY TWENTIETH CENTURY: The British of the early twentieth century found that violet's main values were as a coloring agent and perfume. Because the flowers also possess a gentle laxative quality, a syrup made from them was often recommended for infants.

The rootstocks, on the other hand, were known to be strongly emetic and were occasionally added to more expensive purgative preparations.

For urinary complaints, especially that of gravel, a preparation of the seeds was considered helpful.

Most notable at the time was a preparation of the plant's fresh leaves that was employed both internally and externally to treat cancer. And despite the fact that the journal *British Pharmacopoeia* did not officially approve of the treatment, the publication did include a description of the remedy. Several cases at the time were reported to have been cured with preparations of violet.[570]

Slovaks of the era had a saying to ward off spring colds: "Whoever swallows the first violet flower found in March does not get the fever"; it was said that one did not get a cough either. Slovaks made a healing ointment by filling a bottle with violet leaves, adding olive oil, and leaving the corked bottle in the sun for thirty days. They then strained the mixture through a cloth, rebottling the infused oil for medicinal purposes.[571]

It is also worth noting that, in the late nineteenth century, the popular and well-regarded Bavarian priest Sebastian Kneipp recommended that his many followers take the violet's flowers and leaves as teas, especially for severe coughs and strong headaches.[572]

In Russian folk medicine, decoctions from violets were used as a diuretic, against kidney and bladder stones, rheumatism, lung diseases, bronchitis, and whooping cough. The flowers and roots were also used for coughs and as an expectorant.[573]

VIOLA IN ASHKENAZI HERBALISM IN THE PALE IN THE EARLY TWENTIETH CENTURY: In the presumed existing record of Ashkenazi herbalism in the Pale of Settlement, interpretation of violet's healing virtues diverges a little from the mainstream here. While most of what's been written about the plant's medicinal qualities in the West and Near East are mainly concerned with violet's ability to soothe respiratory afflictions, skin inflammations, headaches, and urinary tract discomforts, little can be found about the plant's affinity for the heart. The closest I've encountered is a brief mention in the Russian literature of violet's support for those who have experienced a heart attack. A possible second explanation for the plant's affinity for the organ may be interpreted in Hildegard von Bingen's observation nearly a thousand years ago in which she connects feelings of sadness with difficulty breathing. It may have been these traditions that healers in the Pale were calling on when they looked to violet as a heart remedy, or even directly back to the ancient Greeks.

In the towns and villages of the Pale, specific species of violet were employed for the treatment of heart disease. None of the healers surveyed between the world wars reported applications of the most common and popular species, *V. odorata*, that was used medicinally in other parts of Europe. Instead, they sought out and relied on the following closely related plants for their remedies.

Viola Mirabilis L. (English: wonder violet; Ukrainian: Фіялка дивовижна, фіялка, сердечник, зозулині черевички, польові лісові калачики, зараза, бишишник; Russian: фиялка удивительная) A decoction or infusion of the whole plant or only the leaves and flowers was used for the treatment of heart trouble, palpitation, and shortness of breath by folk healers in Lachovitz, Polona, Makhnivke, and Barditchev. The remedy book of Yoel Ba'al Shem also summons the root of the violet in his recipe for coughs, shortness of breath, and heart pains.[574]

Viola Hirta L. (English: horse violet, hairy violet; Ukrainian: Фіялка мохната, фіялка волосиста, фіялка, фіялочки, черевички, жирицвіт, мудики; Russian: Фиалка опушённая, или Фиалка коротковолосистая) In Barditchev and Letichev, a decoction of the entire plant including the roots was given in cases of heart trouble and shortness of breath. This remedy is further confirmed by a separate study of the Podolia region that includes Letichev. Descendants of

Letichev's inhabitants note that wild pansy, or *Viola tricolor*, was looked to by community healers as a remedy for heart palpitations and coughs.[575]

Viola Epipsila Ldb. (English: dwarf marsh violet; Ukrainian: фіялка; Russian: Фиалка лысая, Фиалка сверху-голая) A decoction of the plant was given by folk healers for the treatment of heart diseases in the community of Ulanov.

Viola Riviniana Rchb. (English: dog violet; Ukrainian: серечник, золотушник; Russian: Фиалка Ривинуса) In Bazilia traditional healers gave an infusion of the herb's leaves and flowers for the relief of heart pain.[576]

PART III

AFTERWORD

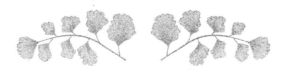

THIS BOOK IS AS MUCH A PIECE OF DETECTIVE work as it is a guide. Throughout the research we conducted, we endlessly ran up against what we called "the
quadruple erasure" of traditional plant and healing knowledge among the Jews
in the Pale of Settlement.

In the early twentieth-century ethnographic work, whether conducted by An-
Sky or by YIVO, women's knowledge was largely written out of the published
record, or when it was included, the researchers emphasized magico-religious
functions (verbal magic). So much of this knowledge is dismissed throughout as
"quackery" or "superstition." The emphasis throughout is largely on the world
of men, and that of observant Jews.

Then there is the work of Soviet plant researchers, as refracted through the
writing of Natalia Ossadcha-Janata, who was circumspect to the point of opacity in identifying the ethnic groups living in the areas where she conducted her
research in the 1920s and 1930s. Whatever the reason for this reticence, the fact
remains that Ossadcha-Janata and her expeditions spent much of their time in
Right Bank Ukraine (Podolia, Volhynia, etc.) in towns and districts that either
had a majority or a plurality Jewish population. No references to Jews appear
in her published work.[1]

And there is the received notion of everyday life in the Jewish settlements
of the Pale, the *shtetlekh* and *derfer,* as a world of markets and shuls, learning
and faith, piety and tradition—a world in which Ashkenazi Jews were embedded

wholly in the realms of the historical, the political, the religious, rather than the natural world, that of animals, seasons, and, most of all, plants. What emerged from our research was a world in which Ashkenazi Jews lived and thrived in the natural world, alongside their non-Jewish neighbors, helping and being helped in turn.

And finally there is the great erasure: the end of communal Jewish life in Eastern Europe during the Shoah.

All of which made for challenges in the research—and continue to make challenges. During the project, we likened the research to peering through a keyhole, not knowing what we were seeing or how it related to something seen through a nearby keyhole.

And this is due primarily to these four erasures, the last of which ensured that the Ashkenazi communities of Eastern Europe (or any Jewish communities throughout most of Europe) would never be able to be studied again *in situ*. They are frozen in time and place, and we rely on the few pieces of research that have come down to us, and we hope that archives as yet unexamined by us may reveal more.

But we have laid the foundation, and we continued to surprise ourselves while putting this book together. The reader will note that the plant uses documented by Natalia Ossadcha-Janata and her expeditions of the late twenties and thirties do not always align with the standard Ukrainian work of Nosal' and Nosal' (Nosal' the elder having also conducted his research into medicinal plant use among Ukrainians in the early twentieth century): we found it significant that *Viburnum opulus*, or guelder rose (Ukrainian *kalyna*), is barely mentioned in her survey, despite the fact that it has well-known healing properties and is also something of a national symbol of Ukraine. In those towns visited by Ossadcha-Janata that had the greatest population percentage of Jews, plant use often harkened back to the tradition of Dioscorides, a tradition often quite distinct from plant uses common to many peoples of Eastern Europe. Does this indicate two distinct but intertwined traditions, possibly demarcated by gender (literate male healers—the ba'alei shem and the feldshers—and female healers such as opshprekherins and midwives)? A review of the plant use documented by Ossadcha-Janata does suggest this.

We do not know how much more information we may be able to find as we continue to explore this topic. There are other plants to discuss, other archives to explore, other leads to follow, other threads to chase. We have tantalizing clues that suggest a Silk Road route by which Eastern plants and plant knowledge were brought to Eastern Europe from Central and East Asia—Jewish communities in the Pale made use of a number of plants unknown to Dioscorides and his successors. We have many more primary sources from the Pale to review, such as Yiddish- and Hebrew-language yizkor books, the vast array of Hebrew *segulot* and *refu'ot* from the eighteenth and nineteenth centuries, and the wilderness of Hebrew plant nomenclature (only partially documented by Immanuel Löw in his four-volume, two-thousand-page *Flora der Juden*). And most interestingly, we suspect that more of the world of women's knowledge and women's medicine is reflected in the written records of the Jewish communities of Eastern Europe than earlier scholars have expected, recognized, or acknowledged.

There are many more Ashkenazi roots to disentangle, and we hope that this book will lead more people to explore this hidden tradition that we think we have revealed just a bit.

What else do we say about method? We went about it as we went along, tracing and tracking. Trained librarians both, we knew how to follow citations and how to read footnotes and endnotes carefully. Gazetteers, maps, dictionaries, piles of books in seven or eight languages (not all of them ones we know well), and just a lot of disentangling—an entire universe of knowledge that had fallen through the cracks. For so many decades, particularly in the late nineteenth and early twentieth centuries (the last period when ethnobotanical research among the Jews of the Pale even could be conducted), scientific progress was dismissive of traditional knowledge; this refusal to take traditional knowledge seriously was most sharply realized in the Pale, among Jewish communities that, lacking sponsored, large-scale organizations that would document and preserve folkways, remained sequestered in ghettos and shtetls or deracinated in the big cities.

But things seep through. Here is an estimable piece of detective work in what we have come to call "the hidden herbal." In the words of Natalia Ossadcha-Janata:

> *In addition to technical difficulties (absence of our own means of transportation, etc.), we were faced with another considerable difficulty, namely the fact that in the Soviet Union the so-called "village quacks," i.e., the persons who applied methods and treatments of folk medicine, were punished*

by imprisonment, and therefore they were afraid to tell about what they were doing. To quote just one example: we met a woman in the Odessa region who was 102 years old, and who treated nervous affections and other diseases by hypnosis and herbs. However, all she would tell us was that she cured her patients with the help of "God's word." Sick people came to see her or were brought to her from places as far as Kharkov, Odessa, and Kiev. A few years earlier she had been ordered to discontinue her treatments, since she had no medical training, and was even arrested. Thanks to the intervention of a local high official whom she had cured, she was released, and even allowed unofficially to continue her treatments. However, afraid of being jailed again, she mentioned only a few of the herbs she was using.[2]

This elder who healed "nervous affections" (*sic*) and other disorders with "hypnosis and herbs" can now be positively identified as a medicine woman, or shamanic healer. On further investigation we can also ascertain that she is the interviewee from the town of Lyubashivka.

In *Herbs Used in Ukrainian Folk Medicine,* only three towns in the "Odessa region" are included in the survey: Savran, Troitske, and Lyubashivka. In Savran and Troitske, healers reported knowledge of sixteen and nineteen herbs, respectively. In Lyubashivka the informant only mentions five plants (*Delphinium consolida, Lavatera thuringiaca, Sedum acre, Urtica urens* [all discussed in the "Materia Medica"], and *Crataegus monogyna,* or hawthorn), which would qualify as a "handful" when compared to the relatively large number of plants reported by healers in the other two locations in the Odessa region. At the time of the surveys, Lyubashivka was mostly Jewish, which suggests that the 102-year-old medicine woman was most likely Jewish, perhaps an opshprekherin. Regardless of her ethnicity, both Jews and non-Jews who practiced healing in this magico-religious way shared their healing techniques with one another.

It's interesting how Ossadcha-Janata reports that patients came from as far as Kharkov, Odessa, and Kiev to see her. Up until the Second World War, all three of these large cities had populations that were mostly Jewish and ethnic Russian (not ethnic Ukrainian). We might speculate that the traveling patients who made their way back to the mostly Jewish town of Lyubashivka would have been one-time residents who had gone off to the big cities but continued to return for familiar traditional healing. Or perhaps her renown was such that patients traveled long distances in search of her remedies.

We hope to review whatever additional archival material may be available in order to more closely interrogate the particulars of these informants from the Soviet Union before the Second World War.

In contemplating (and being frustrated by) the erasures, we call for a recapitulation of healing that will engender a scientific or clinical medicine that is respectful of the traditions that bore it and of those practitioners who continue to work in the traditions. We call for a healing that, instead of exploiting people and plants, honors Indigenous knowledge and the natural world and respects the whole plant as medicine rather than as an assembly of discrete constituents to be extracted.

APPENDIX 1

PALE OF SETTLEMENT TOWNS REFERENCED IN "MATERIA MEDICA" WITH SIGNIFICANT ASHKENAZI POPULATIONS CIRCA 1926

PRE-WW2 YIDDISH LOCATION NAME	PRESENT-DAY NAME	OTHER LOCATION INFORMATION	TOTAL POPULATION (1926, UNLESS OTHERWISE NOTED)	ASHKENAZI POPULATION (1926, UNLESS OTHERWISE NOTED)	PERCENTAGE ASHKENAZI
Anopol	Hannopil	Khmelnytskyi Oblast, Ukraine	1,897	1,259	67.4
Apt	Opatów	Świętokrzyskie Voivodeship, Poland	10,200* (1938)	6,000 (1938)	58.8
Balte	Balta	Odessa Oblast, Ukraine	23,034	9,916	39.6
Barditchev	Berdychiv	Zhytomyr Oblast, Ukraine	55,417	30,812	55.6
Bazilia	Bazaliya	Khmelnytskyi Oblast, Ukraine	3,020	353	11.7
Birzula (Kotovsk after 1935)	Podilsk	Odessa Oblast, Ukraine	10,007	2,507	25
Bohslov	Bohuslav	Kyiv Oblast, Ukraine	12,111	6,432	53
Broslev	Bratslav	Vinnytsia Oblast, Ukraine	7,842	1,840	24.7
Cherkoss	Cherkasy	Cherkasy Oblast, Ukraine	39,511	10,886	28.2
Chopovitch	Chopovychi	Zhytomyr Oblast, Ukraine	9,369	1,533	25
Eishyshok	Eišiškės	Lithuania	2,382 (1921)	687 (1921)	28.8
Khmelnik	Khmilnyk	Vinnytsia Oblast, Ukraine	10,792	6,011	55.6
Kiev	Kyiv	Kyiv Oblast, Ukraine	513,637	140,256	27.3
Kolenivka	Kalynivka	Vinnytsia Oblast, Ukraine	2,418	1,097	41
Konotop	Konotop	Sumy Oblast, Ukraine	33,200	5,763	17
Korosten	Korosten	Zhytomyr Oblast, Ukraine	12,012	6,089	51
Korsn	Korsun-Shevchenkivskyi	Cherkasy Oblast, Ukraine	4,775	2,449	51.2
Kresilev	Krasyliv	Khmelnytskyi Oblast, Ukraine	4,925	1,550	31
Kurenets	Kurenets	Belarus	1,770 (1897)	1,613 (1897)	90.9
Lachovitz	Bilohiria	Khmelnytskyi Oblast, Ukraine	1,581	844	53.4
Ladizhin	Ladyzhyn	Vinnytsia Oblast, Ukraine	6,500 (1897)	3,212 (1897)	49
Letichev	Letychiv	Khmelnytskyi Oblast, Ukraine	7,160	2,434	34
Litin	Lityn	Vinnytsia Oblast, Ukraine	8,382	2,487	30
Lochvitza	Lokhvytsia	Poltava Oblast, Ukraine	10,834	2,095	20
Luben	Lubny	Poltava Oblast, Ukraine	21,302	5,341	25

Lyubashivka	Liubashivka	Odessa Oblast Ukraine	>500 (1939)	671 (1939)	~100
Makhnivka	Makhnivka	Vinnytsia Oblast, Ukraine	5,343 (1897)	2,435 (1897)	45
Maryupol	Mariupol	Donetsk Oblast, Ukraine	63,920	7,332	17.5
Melitopol	Melitopol	Zaporizhia Oblast, Ukraine	25,545	8,583†	33.6
Monasterishtche	Monastyryshche	Cherkasy Oblast, Ukraine	2,045 (1926)	2,620 (1900)	?
Olt-Kosntin	Starokostiantyni	Khmelnytskyi Oblast, Ukraine	16,807	6,934	41.3
Polona	Polonne	Khmelnytskyi Oblast, Ukraine	16,400	5,337	32.5
Priluki	Pryluky	Chernihiv Oblast, Ukraine	28,621	9,001	31.4
Riga	Riga	Latvia	377,917 (1930)	42,328 (1930)	11.2
Ritzev	Hrytsiv	Khmelnytskyi Oblast, Ukraine	4,247	1,578	37
Romen	Romny	Sumy Oblast, Ukraine	25,787	9,747	33
Savran	Savran	Odessa Oblast, Ukraine	8,243	3,198	39
Shepetovka	Shepetivka	Khmelnytskyi Oblast, Ukraine	14,693	3,916	27
Shvarts–Timeh	Bila Tserkva	Kyiv Oblast, Ukraine	42,974	15,624	36.4
Slovita	Slavuta	Khmelnytskyi Oblast, Ukraine	10,478	4,701	44.9
Tchan	Teofipol	Khmelnytskyi Oblast, Ukraine	3,676	1,483	40
Tishevits	Tyszowce	Lublin Voivodeship, Poland	4,420	2,451	55
Ulanov	Ulaniv	Vinnytsia Oblast, Ukraine	2,841	2,151	70.5
Uman	Uman	Kyiv Oblast, Ukraine	44,812	22,179	49.5
Vinitza	Vinnytsia or Vinnytsya or Vinnitsa	Vinnytsia Oblast, Ukraine	58,000	21,812	37.6
Yekaterinoslav	Dnipro	Dnipropetrovsk Oblast, Ukraine	232,925	62,073	26.9
Yelisavetgrod	Kropyvnytskyi	Kirovohrad Oblast, Ukraine	100,331	18,358	27.7
Yozefov	Józefów	Lublin Voivodeship, Poland	1,344 (1921)	1,056 (1921)	79
Zaslov	Iziaslav	Khmelnytskyi Oblast, Ukraine	11,707	3,820	32.6
Zhitomir	Zhytomyr	Zhytomyr Oblast, Ukraine	69,465	29,503 (1939)	40
Zvenigorodka	Zvenyhorodka	Cherkasy Oblast, Ukraine	18,018	6,584	37

Unless otherwise noted, all data is taken from Seltzer, *Columbia Lippincott Gazetteer*; Erenburg and Grossman, *Black Book*; Mokotoff and Sack, *Where Once We Walked*; jewishgen.org and rujen.ru; and various Wikipedia entries.

* From www.encyclopedia.com/religion/encyclopedias-almanacs-transcripts-and-maps/melitopol

† Polish census from: Artur Lis, "Żydzi w Opatowie w XVI-XVIII wieku," *Roczniki Humanistyczne* 58, no. 2 (2010): 95–111.

APPENDIX 2

TIMELINE OF SOURCES REFERRED TO IN TEXT

c. 371–328 BCE Theophrastus Philosopher and close colleague of Aristotle

23/24–79 CE Pliny the Elder (Gaius Plinius Secundus) Roman author, naturalist, and natural philosopher

c. 40–90 Dioscorides (Pedanius Dioscorides) Greek physician, pharmacologist, botanist, and author of *De materia medica*—a five-volume Greek encyclopedia about herbal medicine and related medicinal substances that was widely read for more than 1,500 years

129–200 Galen (Aelius Galenus or Claudius Galenus) Greek surgeon, philosopher, and physician

980–1037 Avicenna (Ibn Sina or Abu Ali Sina, Pur Sina) Persian polymath who is regarded as one of the most significant physicians, astronomers, thinkers, and writers of the Islamic Golden Age, and the father of modern medicine

1098–1179 Hildegaard von Bingen (or Hildegard von Bingen, also known as Saint Hildegard) German Benedictine abbess, herbalist, writer, composer, philosopher, Christian mystic, visionary, and polymath, considered by many to be the founder of scientific natural history in Germany

1135–1204 Moses ben Maimon (commonly known as Maimonides, also referred to by the acronym Rambam) Medieval Sephardic Jewish philosopher, astronomer, and physician

1200–1280 Albertus Magnus German friar, bishop, and alchemist

1493/4–1541 Paracelsus (Philippus Aureolus Theophrastus Bombastus von Hohenheim) Swiss physician, alchemist, lay theologian, and philosopher

1528–1586 Adam Lonicer (Adam Lonitzer or Adamus Lonicerus) German botanist

1540–1611 Simon Syreniusz (or Szymon Syreński) Pre-Linnean Polish botanist who published a botanic atlas in five volumes describing 765 plants

1545–1612 Gerard or John Gerard (also John Gerarde) English botanist and author of the illustrated *Herball, or Generall Historie of Plantes*, first published in 1597

1567–1650 John Parkinson English herbalist, botanist, and apothecary to James I

1616–1654 Nicholas Culpeper English botanist, herbalist, physician, astrologer, and author of *The Complete Herbal*, 1653

1644–1713 William Salmon English empiric doctor and writer of medical texts

1652–1729 Tobias ha-Kohen (also known as Tobiyya/Tuviyah Cohn/Kohn/Kats) Author of *Ma'aseh Toviyah*, "The Work of Tobias," an early modern encyclopedic work devoted to the sciences, covering theology, botany, medicine, and more. The botany section surveys both herbal remedies and medicinal plant nomenclature from the standpoint of a polyglot trained physician who studied and practiced in western, eastern, and southeastern Europe, before moving to Istanbul to serve as a court physician to the Sublime Porte.

1728–1797 Samuel Auguste (Samuel-Auguste) André David Tissot Swiss physician, published *Avis au peuple sur sa santé*, "Advice to the People," in 1761

1740s–? Moyshe Markuse (Moses Marcuse) German physician and author of *Sefer refu'ot, hanikra ezer yisrael*, or *Ezer Yisrael*, published in 1790

1821–1897 Sebastian Kneipp Bavarian priest and one of the forefathers of the naturopathic medicine movement

1854 *King's American Dispensatory* A book covering the herbs worked with in American medical practice, especially by Eclectic medicine practitioners, a botanical school of medicine in the nineteenth to twentieth centuries that included Native American medicinal practices

GLOSSARY

Herbal Preparations

Decoction a method of boiling in water and then reducing down the liquid from plant materials—especially the harder parts such as roots, wood, bark, and seeds—to extract their most concentrated medicinal qualities

Electuary powdered herbs mixed with syrup or honey; consistency can vary depending on ingredients and taste

Hydromel a drink similar to mead made with fermented honey and water

Infusion similar to a tea; plant material is boiled in water in a covered pot (to avoid the evaporation of volatile oils) for a short period of time

Juice chopped fresh plants squeezed to remove juice, then water is added and the material is pressed again to extract water-soluble constituents sensitive to heat. This method is best for preserving the plant's vitamins and minerals, but juice must be taken soon after pressing, before fermentation begins and medicinal qualities erode.

Poultice (or cataplasm) heated bruised or crushed medicinal parts of plant are applied topically to affected skin. Depending on the plant being applied, the poultice may include other materials such as bread, cornmeal, or cloth to help retain heat and moisture or protect the skin from irritation.

Syrup plant material is boiled in a sweet base such as honey until thicker consistency is reached; especially useful for administering medicine to children

Tincture an extract of plant material using an alcohol (vodka, brandy, etc.) to pull out a plant's medicinal properties

Herbal Actions

Anodyne soothes or diminishes pain

Anthelmintic destroys and expels worms in the intestine

Anti-emetic prevents vomiting

Anti-pyretic reduces fever

Anti-scrofulous prevents or impedes scrofula

Aperient mild laxative

Antispasmodic relieves spasms in the smooth muscles

Astringent tones and tightens the body's tissues, lessening secretions

Bechic relieves coughs

Calefacient creates a sensation of warmth

Carminative relieves gas from the intestines

Cholagogue stimulates the discharge of bile

Choleretic supports elimination of bile by the liver creating a greater flow of bile

Cicatrisant heals by promoting the formation of scar tissue

Clyster injection of liquid into the lower bowel by insertion through the rectum

Demulcent soothes irritated tissues, especially mucus membranes

Depurative assists with the cleansing of impurities from the blood or organs

Diaphoretic (or sudorific) promotes perspiration

Diuretic supports increased production and secretion of urine

Drawing helps remove a foreign body such as a splinter from the skin

Ecchymosis "black and blue mark" usually due to the release of blood to affected tissues after an injury

Emetic causes vomiting

Emmenagogue promotes menstrual flow

Emollient softens and smooths externally

Febrifuge reduces or stops fever

Glyster liquid injected into the rectum to empty or cleanse the bowels, provide nutrition, etc.

Haematuria blood in the urine

Haemoptysis spitting of blood; expectoration of blood, or of bloody mucus, etc., from the lungs or bronchi

Hemostatic stops hemorrhage; styptic

Hepatic supportive of the liver and its functions

Hydragogue causes copious watery discharges from the bowels

Menorrhagia menstrual periods characterized by abnormally heavy or prolonged bleeding

Mineralizer refers to beneficial minerals in plants, e.g., silica found in horsetail that adds elasticity to tissues making them strong but not brittle

Nervine supports the nervous system with calming or soothing effect

Oxytocic stimulates contraction of uterine smooth muscle to facilitate or hasten childbirth and to reduce postpartum hemorrhage

Pectoral relieves coughs

Rubefacient material applied as a local irritant to cause dilation of the capillaries and an increase in blood circulation to area

Tonic strengthens or invigorates an organism

Vermifuge destroys and expels worms in the intestine

Vulnerary promotes healing of wounds and injury in body tissues

MEDICAL TERMS

Carbuncle cluster of pus-filled boils caused by bacterial infection, most commonly Staphylococcus; presence of a carbuncle signifies the immune system is active and fighting the infection

Catarrh profuse discharge of mucus from mucus membranes of nose and eyes that generally accompanies a cold

Chilblains red and itching swelling on fingers or toes caused by exposure to cold

Felon an infection of the pad of the finger

Fistula an abnormal connection, usually the result of an injury or surgery, between two body parts, or between an abscess and the skin or another abscess

Fluxes abnormal discharges of blood or other matter from or within the body

Furuncle swelling and inflammation of skin due to infection of a hair follicle; boil

Meteorism distension of the abdomen, especially caused by gas

Pessary object inserted into vagina to provide support to the organ and tissues

Quinsy originally inflammation of (part of) the throat; currently inflammation of the tonsils with pus discharge

Scrofula a condition in which the bacteria that causes tuberculosis creates symptoms outside the lungs, usually as inflamed and irritated lymph nodes in the neck

Strangury slow and painful discharge of urine, usually drop by drop, caused by blockage or irritation at the base of the bladder

MISCELLANEOUS

Eclectic Medicine a branch of American medicine active in the late nineteenth and early twentieth centuries that relied on herbal remedies, many from Native American sources, along with other substances and physical therapy practices

King's American Dispensatory a reference first published in 1854 that covers herbs used in American medical practice, especially by those involved in Eclectic Medicine

NOTES

PART I

1   American Herbalists Guild, "Herbal Medicine Fundamentals,"
    www.americanherbalistsguild.com/herbal-medicine-fundamentals.

2   Zimmels, *Magicians, Theologians and Doctors*, 32.

3   Epstein, "Doctor Spock," 8.

4   Epstein, "Health and Healing," 694.

5   World Health Organization, "Traditional, Complementary and Integrative Medicine,"
    www.who.int/health-topics/traditional-complementary-and-integrative-medicine.

6   Hanchuk, *Word and Wax*, 8.

7   Hanchuk, 5.

8   Hanchuk, 6.

9   Moskalewicz, Caumanns, and Dross, "Jewish–German–Polish," 1.

10 Zimmels, 1.

11 Zimmels, 2.

12 Berger, *Jews and Medicine*, 16.

13 Berger, 14–15.

14 Epstein, "Health and Healing," 695.

15 Petrovsky-Shern, "Ba'alei Shem," 1:99–100.

16 Petrovsky-Shern, "You Will Find It," 15.

17 Petrovsky-Shtern, "Ba'alei Shem," 99–100.

18 Petrovsky-Shtern, "Demons," 1:222–23.

19 Petrovsky-Shern, "You Will Find It," 15. See also Patai, *On Jewish Folklore*, 49–50.

20 Petrovsky-Shtern, 29–33.

21 Petrovsky-Shtern, "Ba'alei Shem," 99.

22 Trachtenberg, *Jewish Magic and Superstition*, 139–40.

23 Petrovsky-Shtern, "Ba'alei Shem," 100.

24 Petrovsky-Shtern, "You Will Find It," 18.

25 Tuszewicki, "German Medicine," 66.

26 Levy, *Planets, Potions, and Parchments*, 71.

27 Petrovsky-Shtern, 18.

28 Epstein, "Dr. Spock," 3.

29 Petrovsky-Shtern, 18.

30 Petrovsky-Shtern, 18–19.

31 Petrovsky-Shtern, "Ba'alei Shem," 100.

32 Petrovsky-Shtern, "You Will Find It," 19.

33 Petrovsky-Shtern, 19.

34 From the 1765 English-language translation of Tissot, available via Project Gutenberg: www.gutenberg.org/files/39044/39044-h/39044-h.htm.

35 Tuszewicki, "German Medicine," 66.

36 Petrovsky-Shtern, "You Will Find It," 43.

37 McGrew, *Encyclopedia of Medical History*, 30–31.

38 Berger, 19.

39 Petrovsky-Shtern, "You Will Find It," 33.

40 Petrovsky-Shtern, 33.

41 Petrovsky-Shtern, 31.

42 Petrovsky-Shtern, 37–38.

43 Petrovsky-Shtern, 35.

44 Kossoy and Ohry, *The Feldshers*, 40–41.

45 Kossoy and Ohry, 27.

46 Kossoy and Ohry, 27.

47 Kossoy and Ohry, 145.

48 Kossoy and Ohry, 39.

49 Suhl, *One Foot in America*, 12–14.

50 Kossoy and Ohry, 39.

51 Kirshenblatt and Kirshenblatt-Gimblett, *They Called Me Mayer July*, 232.

52 Sidel, "Feldshers and 'Feldsherism,'" 934.

53 Kossoy and Ohry, 76.

54 Kossoy and Ohry, 146.

55 Kossoy and Ohry, 133–37.

56 Tuszewicki, "German Medicine," 66.

57 Tuszewicki, 66–67.

58 Kossoy and Ohry, 93.

59 Von Richter, *Geschichte Der Medicin in Russland*, 112–18. Also discussed in Kossoy and Ohry, 85.

60 Pollack, *Jewish Folkways in Germanic Lands*, 127.

61   Ossadcha-Janata, *Herbs Used in Ukrainian Folk Medicine*, 71.

62   Kossoy and Ohry, 94–95; Ossadcha-Janata, 81–83.

63   Epstein, "Dr. Spock," 9.

64   Zinberg, *Berlin Haskalah*, 155.

65   Zinberg, 160.

66   Tusewicki, 66.

67   Epstein, "Health and Healing," 696.

68   Epstein, "Dr. Spock," 14.

69   Epstein, 15.

70   Katsovitsh, *Days of Our Years*, 150.

71   Epstein, "Health and Healing," 697.

72   Kossoy and Ohry, 170.

73   Kossoy and Ohry, 170.

74   Eliach, *There Once Was a World*, 442.

75   Eliach, 442.

76   Epstein, "Health and Healing," 698. See also Rubin, "Healing with Plants," 174.

77   Epstein, 696.

78   Kossoy and Ohry, 98.

79   Kossoy and Ohry, 164.

80   Sidel, 934.

81   Kugelmass and Boyarin, *From a Ruined Garden*, 81.

82   Conroy, *In Health and in Sickness*, 72.

83   Kossoy and Ohry, 164.

84   Chapin and Weinstock, *Road from Letichev*, 1:181.

85   Shandler and Rosen, *Lives Remembered*, 87.

86   Kossoy and Ohry, 175.

87   Kossoy and Ohry, 113.

88   Kossoy and Ohry, 170.

89   Kirshenblatt and Kirshenblatt-Gimblett, 232.

90   Katsovitsh, 57.

91   Katsovitsh, 85.

92   Eliach, 440.

93   Eliach, 440.

94   See von Richter. Most of his three-volume work is a sourcebook documenting the immigration of individual physicians from western Europe to Russia at the invitation of the Russian court.

95   Conroy, 29.

96   Conroy, 34.

97   Conroy, 103.

98   Conroy, 142.

99   Eliach, 440.

100 Eliach, 444.

101 Eliach, 444.

102 Conroy, 320.

103 Conroy, 153.

104 Conroy, 338–39.

105 Chapin and Weinstock, 1:192.

106 Conroy, 339.

107 Ossadcha-Janata, 5.

108 Ossadcha-Janata, 7–8.

109 Deutsch, "An-Sky and the Ethnography," 266.

110 Ehrenreich and English, 3.

111 Kirshenblatt and Kirshenblatt-Gimblett, 234.

112 Chapin and Weinstock, 1:186.

113 Zborowski, Herzog, and Mead, 313.

114 Wengeroff and Magnus, *Memoirs of a Grandmother*, 2:81.

115 Wengeroff and Magnus, 2:79–80. In the interwar Ukrainian surveys, oats were
     described as a nutritional food for convalescents: in Kresilev an informant reported a
     decoction of oats to be drunk for colds (Ossadcha-Janata, 73). While we don't know
     exactly which type of sarsaparilla the midwife used, it's likely to have been *Smilax
     ornata*, or Jamaican sarsaparilla (Greave, 713).

116 Katsovitsh, 146. This is also apparent in the An-Sky questionnaires reproduced in
     Deutsch, *Jewish Dark Continent*.

117 Epstein, "Health and Healing," 697.

118 Balin, "Call to Serve," 133.

119 Balin, 137.

120 Chapin and Weinstock, 1:185.

121 Kossoy and Ohry, 156.

122 Schloff, *Prairie Dogs Weren't Kosher*, 134–35.

123 US Holocaust Memorial Museum, "Jewish DPs Pose with an ORT Representative at
     the Entrance to a Workshop in the Feldafing Displaced Persons Camp" (photograph
     no. 14307), 1946, https://collections.ushmm.org/search/catalog/pa1053780.

124   Avrutin, *Photographing the Jewish Nation*, 106.

125   Zborowski, Herzog, and Mead, 313.

126   Kossoy and Ohry, 162.

127   Beukers and Waale, *Tracing An-Sky*, 13.

128   Avrutin, 106.

129   While An-sky pioneered large-scale ethnographic research of customs, superstitions, beliefs, and folkways of the Ashkenazim, he was not the first. Regina Lilientalowa (born Gitla Eiger), a Polish Jew, was the first scholar to seriously practice Jewish ethnography, with her 1898 "Przesądy żydowskie" [Jewish superstitions]. And throughout the first quarter of the twentieth century, the German rabbi Max Grunwald published a series of collections of Jewish folk beliefs, remedies, and superstitions: *Aus Hausapotheke und Hexenküche* [From the medicine cabinet and the witch's kitchen].

130   The questionnaire is the focus of Deutsch, *Jewish Dark Continent*; see also Safran, *Wandering Soul*.

131   Deutsch, *Jewish Dark Continent*, 117.

132   Deutsch, 64.

133   Roskies and Roskies, *Shtetl Book*, 122.

134   Beukers and Walle, 111.

135   Beukers and Walle, 111.

136   Zinberg, 159.

137   Zimmels, 140.

138   Kugelmass and Boyarin, 94. Personal note: this account stems from the Polish shtetl of Bilguray (Biłgoraj), the next town over from my grandparents' hometown of Yozefov.

139   Kronenberg, *Khurbn Bilguray*, 139–40. The title of the essay is actually "The Feldsher in Biłgoraj," who treated illnesses too serious for the opshprekherin to cure.

140   Hanchuk, 1.

141   Deutsch, 64.

142   Hanchuk, 8. The term *baba* is strongly associated with magical healing powers in the region: Ashkenazi midwives and healers were known as *bobes*, and Eastern European mythology honors the *zlata baba*, the golden woman, a pre-Christian oracle. One Yiddish travelogue offers the claim that the real-life Golda, wife of Sholem ALeichem's Tevye the milkman, was a "golden woman": "The entire village used to go to her for advice. She would help everyone and she also was a healer. She was our best doctor, with her herbal remedies, which she collected in the forest." (Mendele listserv: www.columbia.edu/~jap2220/Arkhiv/vol03%20(1993-4)/vol03096.txt)

143   Hanchuk, 18.

144   Mucz, *Baba's Kitchen Medicines*, 24.

145   See Beukers and Walle, 111.

146   Mucz, 35.

147   Kirshenblatt and Kirshenblatt-Gimblett, 234.

148   Kirshenblatt and Kirshenblatt-Gimblett, 234; Mucz, 13; Abraham Rechtman, who worked on the An-Sky expeditions, has similar descriptions in his account of opsh-prekherins, *Yidishe etnografye un folklor*, 293–99. In an unexpected twist, a cousin of my father's recently wrote to me that his grandmother, my great-grandmother, who was originally from Kiev before immigrating to the United States, took her children, my grandmother among them, to see the opshprekher, Leybele Satanoffsky, when her children were all very young. This folk healer practiced in South Phila-delphia where my grandmother and her siblings were born and raised in the early twentieth century. Satanoffsky was apparently well-known in this community. See Meyers, *Jewish Community of South Philadelphia*, 95.

149   Rechtman, 295. Translated by the authors.

150   Hanchuk, 54.

151   Zinberg, 163; Eliach, 438.

152   Eliach, 437–38.

153   Eliach, 438.

154   Hanchuk, 16. This is also found in contemporary folk medicine in Ukraine; cf. Ganus, M. "Magichni sposoby likuvannia ditei na Slobozhanshchyni" [Magical means of treating children in Slobozhanshchyna], *Visnyk Kharkivs'kogo natsion-al'nogo universytety imeni V. N. Karazina*, 2016, 23, 80–87.

155   Zinberg, 158.

156   Kugelmass and Boyarin, 94.

157   Eliach, 439.

158   Kugelmass and Boyarin, 95. See "Materia Medica" for plants that are remedies for erysipelas, scrofula, etc. The original Yiddish has "dark royz" rather than black.

159   Kotik and Assaf, *Journey to a Nineteenth-Century Shtetl*, 293.

160   Kotik and Assaf, 293.

161   Zimmels, 3.

162   Zborowski, Herzog, and Mead, 326.

163   Kirshenblatt and Kirshenblatt-Gimblett, 194.

164   Kirshenblatt and Kirshenblatt-Gimblett, 196.

165   Deutsch, *Jewish Dark Continent*, 273. See also Pollack, 48–49.

166   Rechtman, 327.

167   Kugelmass and Boyarin, 76.

168   Deutsch, 273; Kirshenblatt and Kirshenblatt-Gimblett, 151. See also Kugelmass and Boyarin, 77.

169   Kugelmass and Boyarin, 77.

170   Kirshenblatt and Kirshenblatt-Gimblett, 151.

171   Claassens, *Mourner, Mother, Midwife*, 26–27.

172   Claassens, 27.

173   Claassens, 27.

174   Currier, *Songsingers' Land*, 48–50.

175   Currier, 48–51

176   Currier, 52–54.

177   See the Peachridge Glass website section devoted to the Kantorowicz family: www .peachridgeglass.com/2013/12/history-of-kantorowicz-family-and-their-factory/.

178   Woodhead, *War Paint*, 25–26.

179   Rubin, 174–75.

180   Schwartz, Joseph, "Tipn un geshtaltn," 264.

181   Kring, I. "Der mames nit-geshribene sefer ha-refu'os," 547–50.

182   From, Leib. "Der doktor un heymishe refu'os," 345.

183   Tsherniak, "Meditsinishe hilf un meditsinishe anshtaltn," 527.

184   Rubin, 175.

Part II

1   Eliach, 440.

Materia Medica

1   Ossadcha-Janata, 71–72.

2   Dioscorides, *De materia medica*, 186. Grieve, *Modern Herbal*, 26.

3   Dioscorides, 186.

4   Everett, *Alphabet of Galen*, 5.

5   Berger and Hildegard, *Hildegard of Bingen*, 106.

6   Berger and Hildegard, 109.

7   Berger and Hildegard, 151.

8   Hildegard, *Hildegard's Healing Plants*, 181.

9   Paracelsus and Waite, *Hermetic and Alchemical Writings*. All citations are from unpaginated Internet Archive edition.

10 Tuviah ha-Rofe (Tobias Cohn), *Ma'aseh Tuviah*, 233.

11 Lust, *Herb Book*, 92.

12 Easley and Horne, *Modern Herbal Dispensatory*, 173.

13 Gladstar, *Herbal Recipes for Vibrant Health*, 309.

14 Lust, 92.

15 Easley and Horne, 173; Mills and Bone, *Principles and Practice of Phytotherapy*, 71.

16 Hoffmann, *Complete Illustrated Holistic Herbal*, 58.

17 Theiss and Theiss, *Family Herbal*, 100.

18 Zevin, Altman, and Zevin, *Russian Herbal*, 24–25.

19 Knab and Knab, *Polish Herbs*, 85.

20 Knab and Knab, 98.

21 Vasiliauskas, *Vaistažolių Galia*, 10.

22 Khalsa and Tierra, *Way of Ayurvedic Herbs*, 87–88.

23 Hovorka and Kronfeld, *Vergleichende Volksmedizin*, 1:11.

24 Grieve, 28.

25 Müller-Dietz and Rintelen, *Arzneipflanzen in Der Sowjetunion*, 1:49.

26 Kirshenblatt and Kirshenblatt-Gimblett, 232.

27 Ossadcha-Janata, 72.

28 Lust, 120; Grieve, 744.

29 Grieve, 744.

30 Riddle, *Contraception and Abortion*, 91–92.

31 Dioscorides, 176–77.

32 Hildegard, 134.

33 Maimonides and Rosner, *Glossary of Drug Names*, 96.

34 Ossadcha-Janata, 82.

35 Wheelwright, *Medicinal Plants and Their History*, 126.

36 Tissot, *Advice to the People*, 266. Citations taken from Internet Archive edition: www.gutenberg.org/files/39044/39044-h/39044-h.htm.

37 Tissot, 597.

38 Tuviah, 279.

39 Lust, 121.

40 Grieve, 184.

41 Zemlinskii, *Lekarstvennye Rasteniia SSSR*, 374.

42 Hovorka and Kronfeld, 2:179.

43 Ossadcha-Janata, 82.

44 The Perfume Society, "Artemisia," www.perfumesociety.org/ingredients-post/artemisia/.

45 Grieve, 859.

46 Ossadcha-Janata, 39.

47 Moldenke and Moldenke, *Plants of the Bible*, 48.

48 Dioscorides, 87.

49 Dioscorides, 87.

50 Vasiliauskas, 30–31.

51 Berger and Hildegard, 109.

52 Berger and Hildegard, 114.

53 Hildegard, 100.

54 Knab and Knab, 173–74.

55 Knab and Knab, 173.

56 Grieve, 357.

57 Tissot, 596.

58 Tissot, 256.

59 Tissot, 598.

60 Tissot, 282.

61 Mentioned in Tuviah, 241, 251, 282, 301, 304.

62 Easley and Horne, 325.

63 Allen and Hatfield, *Medicinal Plants in Folk Tradition*, 300.

64 Knab and Knab, 173.

65 Vasiliauskas, 30.

66 Grieve, 858–60.

67 Hovorka and Kronfeld, 1:449–50.

68 Nosal' and Nosal', *Likars'ki Roslyny*, 34.

69 Hovorka and Kronfeld, 1:449–50.

70 Müller-Dietz and Rintelen, 1:89; Nosal' and Nosal', 34.

71 Unless otherwise noted, refer to Ossadcha-Janata, 40.

72 Ossadcha-Janata, 40.

73 Kirshenblatt and Kirshenblatt-Gimblett, 33, 121, 144.

74 Eliach, 444.

75 Ossadcha-Janata, 40.

76 Grieve, 178.

77 Dioscorides, 170.

78 Everett, 189.

79   Maimonides and Rosner, 165.

80   Hildegard, 128.

81   Grieve, 179.

82   Grieve, 179.

83   Paracelsus, n.p.

84   Tissot, 54.

85   Grieve, 179.

86   Mills and Bone, 335.

87   Tissot, 489–90.

88   Tuviah, 226.

89   Mills and Bone, 335.

90   Lust, 153.

91   Zevin, Altman, and Zevin, 50–51.

92   Allen and Hatfield, 80.

93   Ossadcha-Janata, 89.

94   Zevin, Altman, and Zevin, 50.

95   Müller-Dietz and Rintelen, 2:39; Nosal' and Nosal', 236.

96   Knab and Knab, 100–01; Hovorka and Kronfeld, 1:385–86.

97   Unless otherwise noted, refer to Ossadcha-Janata, 89–90.

98   Cahan, "Simanim un Segulot," 295–97.

99   Ossadcha-Janata, 89–90.

100   Grieve, 197; Lust, 153.

101   Dioscorides, 147.

102   Grieve, 197.

103   Tuviah, 275, 281.

104   Grieve, 197; Maimonides and Rosner, 83.

105   Maimonides and Rosner, 190.

106   Moldenke and Moldenke, 74.

107   Grieve, 197.

108   Grieve, 198.

109   Foster and Hobbs, *Western Medicinal Plants and Herbs*, 216.

110   Foster and Hobbs, 216.

111   Easley and Horne, 120.

112   Foster and Hobbs, 217.

113   Theiss and Theiss, 32, 23.

114   Mills and Bone, 138.

115   Foster and Hobbs, 217.

116   Grieve, 198.

117   Hovorka and Kronfeld, 1:445–46.

118   Grieve, 198.

119   Knab and Knab, 102.

120   Hovorka and Kronfeld, 1:445–46.

121   Hovorka and Kronfeld, 1:445–46.

122   Müller-Dietz and Rintelen, 1:44; Nosal' and Nosal' 48.

123   Unless otherwise noted, refer to Ossadcha-Janata, 53–54.

124   Tuviah, 275.

125   Tuviah, 285.

126   Chapin and Weinstock, 1:232.

127   Lust, 235.

128   Grieve, 421–22.

129   Grieve, 422.

130   Paracelsus, n.p.

131   Lust, 234.

132   Foster and Hobbs, 198.

133   Allen and Hatfield, 211.

134   King, Felter, and Lloyd, *King's American Dispensatory*. See also Henriette's Herbal
       Homepage, "Cynoglossum—Hound's Tongue," www.henriettes-herb.com/eclectic
       /kings/cynoglossum.html.

135   Grieve, 422.

136   Allen and Hatfield, 211.

137   Müller-Dietz and Rintelen, 2:87.

138   Unless otherwise noted, refer to Ossadcha-Janata, 85–86.

139   Lust, 250.

140   Grieve, 464.

141   Dioscorides, 307; Everett, 277.

142   Knab and Knab, 57.

143   Culpeper, *Complete Herbal*, www.bibliomania.com/2/1/66/113/.

144   Lust, 250; Rose, *Herbs & Things*, 74.

145   Rose, 74; Grieve, 464.

146   Hovorka and Kronfeld, 1:362.

147 Knab and Knab, 127.

148 Müller-Dietz and Rintelen, 2:93.

149 Unless otherwise noted, refer to Ossadcha-Janata, 20–21; covered briefly in Osadcha-Ianata, *Likars'ki roslyny*, 12.

150 Lust, 353.

151 Bruton-Seal and Seal, *Backyard Medicine*, 81.

152 Dioscorides, 266.

153 Grieve, 420; Bruton-Seal and Seal, 81.

154 Grieve, 421.

155 Knab and Knab, 122.

156 Knab and Knab, 123.

157 Foster and Hobbs, 371.

158 Easley and Horne, 250, inter alia.

159 Easley and Horne, 250, inter alia.

160 Bruton-Seal and Seal, 82; Lust, 354.

161 Lust, 354.

162 Hoffmann, *Medical Herbalism*, 547.

163 Bruton-Seal and Seal, 81.

164 Mills and Bone, 221.

165 Foster and Hobbs, 371; Mills and Bone, 220.

166 Zevin, Altman, and Zevin, 86–87.

167 Knab and Knab, 97, 122–24.

168 Grieve, 421.

169 Hovorka and Kronfeld, 1:375.

170 Müller-Dietz and Rintelen, 3:26; Nosal' and Nosal', 175.

171 Unless otherwise noted, refer to Ossadcha-Janata, 24; covered briefly in Osadcha-Ianata, *Likars'ki roslyny*, 10–11.

172 Chapin and Weinstock, 1:192–93.

173 Grieve, 525. (Grieve lists the dropwort under the entry for meadowsweet and gives its Latin name as "*Spiraea Filipendula*.")

174 Dioscorides, 234.

175 Everett, 251.

176 Mességué, *Health Secrets*, 188.

177 Lust, 270.

178 Ody, *Complete Medicinal Herbal*, 58; Bruton-Seal and Seal, 96.

179   Mességué, 188.

180   Mességué, 188; Rose, 83.

181   Hoffmann, *Medical Herbalism*, 550.

182   Clevely and Richmond, *New Guide to Herbs*, 88.

183   Allen and Hatfield, 146.

184   Allen and Hatfield, 352.

185   Easley and Horne, 266.

186   Nosal' and Nosal', 53.

187   Zevin, Altman, and Zevin, 103.

188   Katanic et al., "Dropwort," 18.

189   Grieve, 525.

190   Katanic et al., 2.

191   Ossadcha-Janata, 55.

192   Hovorka and Kronfeld, 1:241.

193   Müller-Dietz and Rintelen, 3:65; Zemlinskii, 383.

194   Unless otherwise noted, refer to Ossadcha-Janata, 55–56; covered briefly in Osadcha-Ianata, *Likars'ki roslyny*, 20.

195   Hovorka and Kronfeld, 2:129; Vogl et al., "Ethnopharmacological in vitro Studies," 751.

196   Chapin and Weinstock, 1:185.

197   Ossadcha-Janata, 63.

198   Lust, 400.

199   Lust, 620.

200   Hildegard, 147.

201   Tuviah, 305.

202   Tuviah, 287.

203   Knab and Knab, 164.

204   Lust, 400.

205   Foster and Hobbs, 44.

206   Allen and Hatfield, 146.

207   Knab and Knab, 164.

208   Lektrava, "Земляника лесная (Fragaria vesca L.)," www.lektrava.ru/encyclopedia /zemlyanika-lesnaya/.

209   Vasiliauskas, 68.

210   Grieve, 777.

211   Hovorka and Fronfeld, 2:420.

212   Hovorka and Kronfeld, 1:125–26; 2:94–95.

213   Müller-Dietz and Rintelen, 3:70.

214   Nosal' and Nosal', 54–56.

215   Unless otherwise noted, refer to Ossadcha-Janata, 67.

216   Lust, 344, Grieve 708.

217   Grieve, 708.

218   Mamedov, Mehdiyeva, and Craker, "Traditional Medicine of the Caucasus," 50.

219   Dioscorides, 247.

220   Everett, 379.

221   Hildegard, 179.

222   Maimonides and Rosner, 84.

223   Moldenke and Moldenke, 43.

224   Paracelsus, n.p.

225   Tuviah, 251, 241.

226   Knab and Knab, 158.

227   Mamedov, Mehdiyeva, and Craker, 50.

228   Mamedov, Mehdiyeva, and Craker, 50.

229   Zevin, Altman, and Zevin, 137.

230   Mamedov, Mehdiyeva, and Craker, 50.

231   Vasiliauskas, 25.

232   Easley and Horn, 307.

233   Gladstar, 360.

234   Hovorka and Kronfeld, 1:230.

235   Knab and Knab, 158.

236   Inventory derived from Nosal' and Nosal', Hovorka and Kronfeld, and Zevin, Altman, and Zevin.

237   Müller-Dietz and Rintelen, 3:135; Zemlinskii, 120.

238   Nosal' and Nosal', 68.

239   Unless otherwise noted, refer to Ossadcha-Janata, 50–52.

240   Chapin and Weinstock, 1:192–93.

241   Kugelmass and Boyarin, 94.

242   Ossadcha-Janata, 52.

243   Ossadcha-Janata, 67; Mességué, 177. See also Annenkov, *Botanicheskii slovar'*, which asserts that the properties of this plant are "like those of Althaea."

244 Grieve, 507; The Lavatera Pages, "Herbaceous Lavateras," www.malvaceae.info /Genera/Lavatera/herbaceous.html#thuringiaca.

245 Dioscorides, 244–45.

246 Everett, 251.

247 Hildegard, 131.

248 Maimonides and Rosner, 279.

249 Tuviah, 235–36, 249, 252, 282–83, 279.

250 Tissot, 277, 308, 369, 375, 412.

251 Tissot, 436, 527.

252 Gladstar, 349.

253 Allen and Hatfield, 108–09.

254 Mills and Bone, 630.

255 Knab and Knab, 137.

256 Zevin, Altman, and Zevin, 26–27.

257 Theiss and Theiss, 78.

258 Müller-Dietz and Rintelen, 4:26; Zemlinskii, 452.

259 Grieve, 507.

260 Knab and Knab, 137.

261 Knab and Knab, 147.

262 Unless otherwise noted, refer to Ossadcha-Janata, 67; covered briefly in Osadcha-Ianata, *Likars'ki roslyny*, 22.

263 Chapin and Weinstock, 1:192–93.

264 Hovorka and Kronfeld, 1:111.

265 Native Plant Trust, "Lepidium ruderale (Stinking Pepperweed)," https://gobotany .nativeplanttrust.org/species/lepidium/ruderale/; NatureGate, "Narrow-leaved Pepperwort," www.luontoportti.com/suomi/en/kukkakasvit/narrow-leaved-pepperwort.

266 Dioscorides, 167.

267 Dioscorides, 167.

268 Maimonides and Rosner, 118.

269 Allen and Hatfield, 120.

270 Bremness, *Complete Book of Herbs*, 136.

271 Easley and Horne, 264.

272 Kim et al., "Anti-Asthmatic Effects," n.p.

273 Reid, *Chinese Herbal Medicine*, 140.

274 Wu, *Illustrated Chinese Materia Medica*, 374.

275 Wheelwright, 164.

276 Foster and Hobbs, 36.

277 Müller-Dietz and Rintelen, 4:36.

278 Unless otherwise noted, refer to Ossadcha-Janata, 41–42; covered briefly in Osadcha-Ianata, *Likars'ki roslyny*, 15–16.

279 Grieve, 592.

280 Lust, 294.

281 Leyel, *Herbal Delights*, 324.

282 Warburg, *Die Muskatnuss*, 9–20.

283 Maimonides and Rosner, 57.

284 Warburg, 33–34.

285 Hildegard, 24–25.

286 Berger and Hildegard, 107.

287 Chevallier, *Encyclopedia of Herbal Medicine*, 115.

288 Warburg, 35–43.

289 Paracelsus, n.p.

290 Tuviah, 287, 215, 234.

291 Leyel, 324.

292 Khalsa and Tierra, 164–67.

293 Chevallier, 115.

294 Rose, 79; Lust, 565.

295 Theiss and Theis, 247.

296 Grieve, 591.

297 Wood et al., *Dispensatory*. All references (unpaginated) are taken from Henriette's Herbal Homepage, www.henriettes-herb.com/eclectic/usdisp/index.html.

298 Hovorka and Kronfeld, 2:134.

299 Leyel, 324.

300 Leyel, 324.

301 Wengeroff, 2:89

302 NatureGate, "White Water-lily," www.luontoportti.com/suomi/en/kukkakasvit/white-water-lily.

303 Tuviah, 290, 303.

304 Petrovsky-Shtern, "You Will Find It," 15.

305 Dioscorides, 238.

306 Maimonides and Rosner, 171.

307 Lektrava, "Кувшинка белая (Nymphaea alba)," www.lektrava.ru/encyclopedia /kuvshinka-belaya/.

308 Lektrava, www.lektrava.ru/encyclopedia/kuvshinka-belaya/.

309 Chevallier, 240.

310 Chevallier, 240.

311 Lektrava, www.lektrava.ru/encyclopedia/kuvshinka-belaya/.

312 Ossadcha-Janata, 12.

313 Müller-Dietz and Rintelen, 4:76.

314 Keller, *Dikie s"edobnye rasteniia*, 7–8.

315 Grieve, 484.

316 Unless otherwise noted, refer to Ossadcha-Janata, 11–13; covered briefly in Osadcha-Ianata, *Likars'ki roslyny*, 7.

317 Lust, 305.

318 Grieve, 606.

319 Ody, 83.

320 Dioscorides, 242.

321 Hildegard, 120.

322 Maimonides and Rosner, 204.

323 Rose, 95.

324 Knab and Knab, 59.

325 Tuviah, 285, 226.

326 Lust, 305.

327 Reid, 97.

328 Ody, 83.

329 Ody, 83.

330 Easley and Horne, 282.

331 Hoffmann, *Medical Herbalism*, 396.

332 Foster and Hobbs, 179.

333 Grieve, 607.

334 Hovorka and Kronfeld, 1:349–50.

335 Ossadcha-Janata, 21.

336 Müller-Dietz and Rintelen, 5:5; Zemlinskii, 422.

337 Unless otherwise noted, refer to Ossadcha-Janata, 22; covered briefly in Osadcha-Ianata, *Likars'ki roslyny*, 12.

338 Bruton-Seal and Seal, 127.

339 Lust, 311.

340 Bruton-Seal and Seal, 127.

341 Dioscorides, 144.

342 Everett, 313.

343 Maimonides and Rosner, 148.

344 Berger and Hildegard, 116.

345 Hildegard, 94.

346 Bruton-Seal and Seal, 127.

347 Tuviah, 234, 247, 252, 216.

348 Tissot, 335.

349 Bruton-Seal and Seal, 128.

350 Lust, 311.

351 Rose, 98.

352 Lust, 311.

353 Hoffmann, *Complete Illustrated Holistic Herbal*, 174.

354 Gladstar, 357.

355 Easley and Horne, 285.

356 Mills and Bone, 209, 211.

357 Bruton-Seal and Seal, 127.

358 Greave, 640.

359 Allen and Hatfield, 247–48.

360 Knab and Knab, 148–49.

361 Zevin, Altman, and Zevin, 118–19.

362 Vasiliauskas, 21.

363 Grieve, 640.

364 Hovorka and Kronfeld, 1:444–45.

365 Knab and Knab, 148-49.

366 Zemlinskii, 214; Nosal' and Nosal', 93–94.

367 Mueller-Dietz and Rintelen, 5:46.

368 Unless otherwise noted, refer to Ossadcha-Janata, 80–81.

369 Chapin and Weinstock, 1:192–93.

370 Trachtenberg, 207.

371 Grieve, 457.

372 Grieve, 457.

373 Dioscorides, 251.

374 Grieve, 457.

375 Ossadcha-Janata, 26; Zevin, Altman, and Zevin, 93.

376 Paracelsus, n.p.

377 Zevin, Altman, and Zevin, 92.

378 Knab and Knab, 72.

379 Lust, 245; Foster and Hobbs, 235.

380 Rose, 104.

381 Foster and Hobbs, 235.

382 Theiss and Theiss, 82.

383 Zevin, Altman, and Zevin, 92–93.

384 Grieve, 458; Allen and Hatfield, 95.

385 Ossadcha-Janata, 26; US Patent Office, "Paul Homero, of Triesta, Austria-Hungary: Medicinal Tea," 1886, https://patentimages.storage.googleapis.com/97/91/f 1/e69e196637d598/US333632.pdf.

386 Ossadcha-Janata, 26.

387 Zemlinskii, 444; Müller-Dietz and Rintelen, 5:56.

388 Nosal' and Nosal', 95.

389 Unless otherwise noted, refer to Ossadcha-Janata, 26–27; covered briefly in Osadcha-Ianata, *Likars'ki roslyny*, 11.

390 Kirshenblatt and Kirshenblatt-Gimblett, 240.

391 Grieve, 740; Lust, 157.

392 Dioscorides, 265.

393 Grieve, 740.

394 Grieve, 740.

395 Hildegard, 50.

396 Maimonides and Rosner, 176.

397 Culpeper, n.p.

398 Tuviah, 291, 296, 298.

399 Knab and Knab, 162.

400 Ossadcha-Janata, 61.

401 Knab and Knab, 162.

402 Zevin, Altman, and Zevin, 53.

403 Lust, 157.

404 Zevin, Altman, and Zevin, 53.

405 Zevin, Altman, and Zevin, 53.

406 Hoffmann, *Complete Illustrated Holistic Herbal*, 127.

407 Foster and Hobbs, 113.

408 Foster and Hobbs, 114.

409 Allen and Hatfield, 142.

410 Allen and Hatfield, 144.

411 Zevin, Altman, and Zevin, 53–54.

412 Grieve, 740–741.

413 Hovorka and Kronfeld, 1:174–75.

414 Ossadcha-Janata, 61–62.

415 Zemlinskii, 386.

416 Unless otherwise noted, refer to Ossadcha-Janata, 62; covered briefly in Osadcha-Ianata, *Likars'ki roslyny*, 20.

417 Lust, 295–96.

418 Grieve, 594–95.

419 Moldenke and Moldenke, 195.

420 Lehner and Lehner, *Folklore and Symbolism,* 42.

421 Moldenke and Moldenke, 195.

422 Grieve, 594.

423 Grieve, 595.

424 Dioscorides, 76.

425 Dioscorides, 77.

426 Maimonides and Rosner, 198.

427 Toviyah, 249.

428 Tissot, n.p.

429 Kirshenblatt and Kirshenblatt-Gimblett, 18.

430 Knab and Knab, 144.

431 Zevin, Altman, and Zevin, 108; Grieve, 594.

432 Lust, 296.

433 Rose, 88–89.

434 Easley and Horn, 319.

435 Allen and Hatfield, 87–88, 355.

436 Ody, 181.

437 Allen and Hatfield, 88.

438 Zevin, Altman, and Zevin, 108–09.

439 Grieve, 595.

440   Knab and Knab, 144.

441   Hovorka and Kronfeld, 2:134.

442   Müller-Dietz and Rintelen 5:83; Zemlinskii, 104; Nosal' and Nosal', 104.

443   Unless otherwise noted, refer to Ossadcha-Janata, 91.

444   Lust, 329.

445   Dioscorides, 263.

446   Tissot, 64.

447   Lust, 369.

448   Allen and Hatfield, 141.

449   Theiss and Theiss, 244.

450   Knab and Knab, 151.

451   Zevin, Altman, and Zevin, 120–21.

452   Vasiliauskas, 11–13.

453   Grieve, 671.

454   Hovorka and Kronfeld, 1:212.

455   Müller-Dietz and Rintelen, 5:105; Zemlinskii, 180.

456   Lewando, *Vilna Vegetarian Cookbook*, 176.

457   Roskies and Roskies, 122.

458   Roskies and Roskies, 307.

459   Eliach, 444.

460   Zborowski, Herzog, and Mead, 196.

461   Kugelmass and Boyarin, 27.

462   Kirshenblatt and Kirshenblatt-Gimblett, 182.

463   Clevely and Richmond, 114.

464   Grieve, 772.

465   Dioscorides, 285.

466   Maimonides and Rosner, 117.

467   Grieve, 772.

468   Ossadcha-Janata, 43.

469   Knab and Knab, 171.

470   Allen and Hatfield, 138–39.

471   Clevely and Richmond, 114.

472   Foster and Hobbs, 106.

473   Wood et al., n.p.

474   Grieve, 772.

475 Clevely and Richmond, 114.

476 Müller-Dietz and Rintelen, 6:34; Zemlinskii, 414.

477 Unless otherwise noted, refer to Ossadcha-Janata, 42–43; covered briefly in Osadcha-Ianata, *Likars'ki roslyny*, 8, 16.

478 Lust, 162.

479 Grieve, 255.

480 Hildegard, 133.

481 Grieve, 218.

482 Paracelsus, n.p.

483 Lust, 162.

484 Ody, 101.

485 Rose, 53.

486 Hoffmann, *Medical Herbalism*, 586.

487 Gladstar, 325.

488 Easley and Horne, 216.

489 Mills and Bone, 148.

490 Allen and Hatfield, 92.

491 Allen and Hatfield, 208.

492 Theiss and Theiss, 256.

493 Knab and Knab, 103–04.

494 Zevin, Altman, and Zevin, 60–61.

495 Grieve, 218.

496 Schulz, *Vorlesungen über Wirkung*, 214; Ossadcha-Janata, 67.

497 Müller-Dietz and Rintelen, 6:69; Zemlinskii, 408; Nosal' and Nosal', 122.

498 Zemlinskii, 408.

499 Unless otherwise noted, refer to Ossadcha-Janata, 77–79.

500 Chapin and Weinstock, 1:193.

501 Grieve, 206, Lust, 394.

502 Ody, 105.

503 Hildegard, 100.

504 Maimonides and Rosner, 243.

505 Allen and Hatfield, 162.

506 Tuviah, 279.

507 Ody, 105.

508 Allen and Hatfield, 162.

509   Mills and Bone, 148, 254, 158, 67.

510   Foster and Hobbs, 160.

511   Rose, 52.

512   Lust, 566.

513   Hoffmann, *Complete Illustrated Holistic Herbal*, 154.

514   Clevely and Richmond, 119.

515   Easley and Horne, 292.

516   Zevin, Altman, and Zevin, 57–58.

517   Knab and Knab, 86.

518   Wood et al., n.p.; Ossadcha-Janata, 30.

519   Grieve, 208; Ody, 105.

520   Müller-Dietz and Rintelen, 7:31; Zemlinskii, 136.

521   Müller-Dietz and Rintelen, 7:31.

522   Ossadcha-Janata, 30.

523   Clevely and Richmond, 119; Lust, 566.

524   Allen and Hatfield, 161.

525   Müller-Dietz and Rintelen, 7:31; Zemlinskii, 137.

526   In Osadcha-Ianata, *Ukraïns'ki narodni nazvy roslyn*, the author also records the Moldovan name "огірочки пэпэнаш" in Kotovs'k.

527   Ossadcha-Janata, 29–34; also covered in briefer detail in Osadcha-Ianata, *Likars'ki roslyny*, 14.

528   Lust, 291.

529   Bruton-Seal and Seal, 114.

530   Moldenke and Moldenke, 237.

531   Dioscorides, 286.

532   Everett, 369.

533   Hildegard, 93.

534   Maimonides and Rosner, 13.

535   Knab and Knab, 142.

536   Zevin, Altman, and Zevin, 106.

537   Rose, 88.

538   Lust, 291; Bruton-Seal and Seal, 114.

539   Mességué, 205.

540   Hoffmann, *Medical Herbalism*, 591; Bruton-Seal and Seal, 114.

541   Gladstar, 353.

542   Bruton-Seal and Seal, 114.

543   Bruton-Seal and Seal, 114.

544   Mességué, 207.

545   Hoffmann, *Medical Herbalism*, 591.

546   Gladstar, 353.

547   Mills and Bone, 490.

548   Hoffmann, *Medical Herbalism*, 591; Mills and Bone, 490; Bruton-Seal and Seal, 114; Foster and Hobbs, 242; Gladstar, 353–54; Mességué, 206–08.

549   Zevin, Altman, and Zevin, 105–06.

550   Vasiliauskas, 19.

551   Grieve, 579.

552   Ossadcha-Janata, 68; Grieve, 578.

553   Hovorka and Kronfeld, 1:89–90.

554   Müller-Dietz and Rintelen, 7:30; Zemlinskii, 150.

555   Ossadcha-Janata, 68-69; also mentioned in Osadcha-Ianata, *Likars'ki roslyny*, 22.

556   Lust, 203; Grieve, 834.

557   Grieve, 834.

558   Grieve, 835.

559   Dioscorides, 295.

560   Mességué, 287; Foster and Hobbs, 216.

561   Hildegard, 96.

562   Culpeper, n.p.

563   Tuviah, 251, 285, 278.

564   Lust, 204.

565   Easley and Horne, 308.

566   Allen and Hatfield, 112.

567   Theiss and Theiss, 133.

568   Knab and Knab, 170.

569   Zevin, Altman, and Zevin, 110.

570   Grieve, 839.

571   Hovorka and Kronfeld, 1:431–32.

572   Knab and Knab, 170.

573   Müller-Dietz and Rintelen, 7:62; Zemlinskii, 451.

574   Ba'al Shem, Katz, and Saye, "Medical Excerpts," 304.

575   Chapin and Weinstock, 1:192–93.

576   Ossadcha-Janata, 18-19.

PART III

1   In her late work, *Ukraïns'ki narodni nazvy roslyn*, Ossadcha-Janata devotes a chapter to foreign (non-Ukrainian) plant names of the region, which includes Bulgarian, Greek, Moldovan, Russian, Tatar, and Czech names, but not Yiddish.

2   Ossadcha-Janata, *Herbs Used in Ukrainian Folk Medicine*, 9.

BIBLIOGRAPHY

Allen, David Elliston, and Gabrielle Hatfield. *Medicinal Plants in Folk Tradition: An Ethnobotany of Britain & Ireland.* Portland, OR: Timber Press, 2004.

Annenkov, N. *Botanicheskii slovar'* [Botanical dictionary]. Sankt-Peterburg, 1878.

Avrutin, Eugene M. *Photographing the Jewish Nation: Pictures from S. An-Sky's Ethnographic Expeditions.* Waltham, MA: Brandeis University Press, 2009.

Ba'al Shem, Yoel, Naphtali Katz, and Hymen Saye. "Medical Excerpts from Sefer Mif'alot Elokim (The Book of God's Deeds)." *Bulletin of the Institute of the History of Medicine* 4, no. 4 (1936): 299–331. www.jstor.org/stable/44438347.

Balin, Carole B. "The Call to Serve: Jewish Women Medical Students in Russia, 1872–1887." In *Jewish Women in Eastern Europe,* edited by Chaeran Freeze, Paula Hyman, and Antony Polonsky, 133–52. Polin: Studies in Polish Jewry, 18. Oxford, UK: Littman Library of Jewish Civilization, 2005.

Berger, Margaret, and Hildegard. *Hildegard of Bingen: On Natural Philosophy and Medicine: Selections from* Cause Et Cure. Library of Medieval Women. Cambridge, UK: D. S. Brewer, 1999.

Berger, Natalia. *Jews and Medicine: Religion, Culture, Science.* Philadelphia: The Jewish Publication Society, 1995.

Beukers, Mariella, and Renée Waale. *Tracing An-Sky: Jewish Collections from the State Ethnographic Museum in St. Petersburg.* Zwolle, Netherlands: Waanders, 1992.

Branover, Herman, ed. *Rossiiskaia Evreiskaia Entsiklopediia* [Russian Jewish encyclopedia]. Moskva: RAEN, 1994. www.rujen.ru.

Bremness, Lesley. *The Complete Book of Herbs.* New York: Viking Studio Books, 1988.

Bruton-Seal, Julie, and Matthew Seal. *Backyard Medicine: Harvest and Make Your Own Herbal Remedies.* New York: Castle Books, 2012.

Cahan, Y. L. "Simanim un Segulot vegn Beli-kheym un Geviksn" [Signs and remedies involving animals and plants]. In *Yidisher folklor. Shriftn fun Yidishn Yivsnshaftlekhn Institut,* Bd. 9, 277–97. Vilne: YIVO, 1938.

Chapin, David A., and Ben Weinstock. *The Road from Letichev: The History and Culture of a Forgotten Jewish Community in Eastern Europe.* 2 vols. San Jose, CA: Writer's Showcase, 2000.

Chevallier, Andrew. *Encyclopedia of Herbal Medicine.* 3rd American ed. New York: DK Publishing, 2016.

Claassens, Juliana M. *Mourner, Mother, Midwife: Reimagining God's Delivering Presence in the Old Testament.* Louisville, KY: Westminster John Knox Press, 2012.

Clevely, A. M., and Katherine Richmond. *The New Guide to Herbs.* London: Lorenz, 1999.

Conroy, Mary Schaeffer. *In Health and in Sickness: Pharmacy, Pharmacists, and the Pharmaceutical Industry in Late Imperial, Early Soviet Russia.* East European Monographs, No. 386. Boulder, CO: East European Monographs, 1994.

Culpeper, Nicholas. *The Complete Herbal.* First published 1653. www.bibliomania .com/2/1/66/113/.

Currier, Alvin C. *The Songsingers' Land and the Land of Mary's Song: An Introduction to (and Meditation on) Karelian Orthodox Culture.* Colfax, WI: A. C. Currier, 1991.

Deutsch, Nathaniel. "An-Sky and the Ethnography of Jewish Women." In *The Worlds of S. An-Sky: A Russian Jewish Intellectual at the Turn of the Century,* edited by Gabriella Safran and Steven J. Zipperstein, 266–79. Stanford, CA: Stanford University Press, 2006.

Deutsch, Nathaniel. *The Jewish Dark Continent: Life and Death in the Russian Pale of Settlement.* Cambridge, MA: Harvard University Press, 2011.

Dioscorides Pedanius. *De materia medica.* Translated by Lily Y. Beck. Altertumswissenschaftliche Texte Und Studien, Bd. 38. Hildesheim, Germany: Olms-Weidmann, 2017.

Easley, Thomas, and Steven H. Horne. *The Modern Herbal Dispensatory: A Medicine-Making Guide.* Berkeley, CA: North Atlantic Books, 2016.

Ehrenreich, Barbara, and Deirdre English. *Witches, Midwives, and Nurses: A History of Women Healers.* Detroit: Black & Red, 1973.

Eliach, Yaffa. *There Once Was a World: A Nine-Hundred-Year Chronicle of the Shtetl of Eishyshok.* Boston: Little, Brown, 1998.

Epstein, Lisa. "Doctor Spock for the 1890s: Medical Advice Literature for Jews of the Russian Empire." *Shofar* 17, no. 4 (Summer 1999): 1–19. www.doi.org/10.1353/sho.1999.0083.

Epstein, Lisa. "Health and Healing." In *YIVO Encyclopedia of Jews in Eastern Europe,* edited by Gershon David Hundert, 694–98. 2 vols. New York: YIVO Institute for Jewish Research, 2010.

Erenburg, Il'ia, and Vasilii Semenovich Grossman. *The Black Book: The Ruthless Murder of Jews by German-Fascist Invaders throughout the Temporarily-Occupied Regions of the Soviet Union and in the Death Camps of Poland during the War of 1941–1945.* New York: Holocaust Publications, 1981.

Everett, Nicholas. *The Alphabet of Galen: Pharmacy from Antiquity to the Middle Ages: A Critical Edition of the Latin Text with English Translation and Commentary.* Toronto: University of Toronto Press, 2012.

Foster, Steven, and Christopher Hobbs. *A Field Guide to Western Medicinal Plants and Herbs.* Peterson Field Guide Series. Boston: Houghton Mifflin, 2002.

From, Leyb. "Der doktor un heymishe refuos" [The doctor and domestic remedies]. *Sefer Zikaron Voislavitsa*. Tel Aviv: Irgun yot'se Vislavitsah be-Yisrael, 1970, 344–46. https://digitalcollections.nypl.org/items/9ef15440-4df7-0134-0d8b-00505686a51c.

Gladstar, Rosemary. *Rosemary Gladstar's Herbal Recipes for Vibrant Health: 175 Teas, Tonics, Oils, Salves, Tinctures, and Other Natural Remedies for the Entire Family.* North Adams, MA: Storey, 2008.

Grieve, Maude. *A Modern Herbal: The Medicinal, Culinary, Cosmetic and Economic Properties, Cultivation and Folk-Lore of Herbs, Grasses, Fungi, Shrubs, and Trees with All Their Modern Scientific Uses.* 2 vols. 1931. Reprint, New York: Dover, 1971.

Hanchuk, Rena Jeanne. *The Word and Wax: A Medical Folk Ritual among Ukrainians in Alberta.* Edmonton: Canadian Institute of Ukrainian Studies Press, 1999.

Hildegard. *Hildegard's Healing Plants: From Her Medieval Classic Physica.* Boston: Beacon Press, 2001.

Hoffmann, David. *The Complete Illustrated Holistic Herbal: A Safe and Practical Guide to Making and Using Herbal Remedies.* Shattesbury, UK: Element Books, 1996.

Hoffmann, David. *Medical Herbalism: The Science and Practice of Herbal Medicine.* Rochester, VT: Healing Arts Press, 2003.

Hovorka, Oskar, and Adolf Kronfeld. *Vergleichende Volksmedizin: Eine Darstellung Volksmedizinischer Sitten Und Gebräuche, Anschauungen Und Heilfaktoren, Des Aberglaubens Und Der Zaubermedizin* [Comparative folk medicine: an overview of folk medicinal customs and practices, attitudes, and cures, superstitions, and magical medicine]. 2 vols. Stuttgart, Germany: Strecker & Schröder, 1908.

JewishGen Communities Database and JewishGen Gazetteer. www.jewishgen.org.

Katanic, Jelena, Vladimir Mihailovic, Nevena Stankovic, Tatjana Boroja, Milan Mladenovic, Slavica Solujic, Milan S. Stankovic, and Miroslav M. Vrvic. "Dropwort (*Filipendula hexapetala* Gilib.): Potential Role as Antioxidant and Antimicrobial Agent." *EXCLI Journal* 14 (2015): 1–20. www.doi.org/10.17179/excli2014-479.

Katsovitsh Yisrael Iser. *The Days of Our Years: Personal and General Reminiscence (1859–1929).* Translated by Maximilian Hurwitz. New York: Jordan, 1929.

Keller, B. A., ed. *Dikie s"edobnye rasteniia* [Wild edible plants]. Moskva, Leningrad: Izd-vo AN SSSR, 1941.

Khalsa, Karta Purkh Singh, and Michael Tierra. *The Way of Ayurvedic Herbs: The Most Complete Guide to Natural Healing and Health with Traditional Ayurvedic Herbalism.* Twin Lakes, WI: Lotus, 2008.

Kim, Sung-Bae, Yun-Soo Seo, Hyo Seon Kim, A. Yeong Lee, Jin Mi Chun, Byeong Cheol Moon, and Bo-In Kwon. "Anti-Asthmatic Effects of Lepidii seu Descurainiae Semen Plant Species in Ovalbumin-Induced Asthmatic Mice." *Journal of Ethnopharmacology* 244 (2019): 112083. www.doi.org/10.1016/j.jep.2019.112083.

King, John, Harvey Wickes Felter, and John Uri Lloyd. *King's American Dispensatory*. 19th ed., 3rd rev. ed. Cincinnati: Ohio Valley, 1905.

Kirshenblatt, Mayer, and Barbara Kirshenblatt-Gimblett. *They Called Me Mayer July: Painted Memories of a Jewish Childhood in Poland before the Holocaust*. Berkeley: University of California Press, 2007.

Knab, Sophie Hodorowicz, and Mary Anne Knab. *Polish Herbs, Flowers and Folk Medicine*. Rev. ed. New York: Hippocrene Books, 1999.

Kossoy, Edward, and Abraham Ohry. *The Feldshers: Medical, Sociological and Historical Aspects of Practitioners of Medicine with Below University Level Education*. Jerusalem: Magnes Press, 1992.

Kotik, Yekhezhel, and David Assaf. *Journey to a Nineteenth-Century Shtetl: The Memoirs of Yekhezkel Kotik*. Raphael Patai Series in Jewish Folklore and Anthropology. Detroit: Wayne State University Press in cooperation with the Diaspora Research Institute, Tel Aviv University, 2002.

Kring, I. "Der mames nit-geshribener sefer ha-refu'os" [Mama's unwritten book of remedies]. *Felshṭin: zamlbukh tsum ondenḳ fun di Felshtiner ḳedoyshim*. First Felshteener Benevolent Association. Nyu Yorḳ: Aroysgegebn fun Felshṭiner fareyn, 1937, 547–62. www .yiddishbookcenter.org/collections/yizkor-books/yzk-nybc313760/.

Kronenberg, Avraham. *Khurbn Bilguray* [The destruction of Biłgoraj]. Tel Aviv: Irgun Yots'e Bilgoray, 716, [1955 or 1956]. www.yiddishbookcenter.org/collections/yizkor-books /yzk-nybc317983.

Kugelmass, Jack, and Jonathan Boyarin. *From a Ruined Garden: The Memorial Books of Polish Jewry*. New York: Schocken Books, 1983.

Lehner, Ernst, and Johanna Lehner. *Folklore and Symbolism of Flowers, Plants and Trees*. New York: Tudor, 1960.

Levy, B. Barry. *Planets, Potions, and Parchments: Scientifica Hebraica from the Dead Sea Scrolls to the Eighteenth Century*. Montreal: McGill-Queen's University Press, 1990.

Lewando, Fania. *The Vilna Vegetarian Cookbook*. Translated by Eve Jochnowitz. New York: Schocken Books, 2015.

Leyel, C. F. *Herbal Delights: Tisanes, Syrups, Confections, Electuaries, Robs, Juleps, Vinegars, and Conserves*. Boston: Houghton Mifflin, 1938.

Lust, John B. *The Herb Book*. New York: Bantam Books, 1974.

Maimonides, Moses, and Fred Rosner. *Moses Maimonides' Glossary of Drug Names*. Memoirs of the American Philosophical Society, Vol. 135. Philadelphia: American Philosophical Society, 1979.

Mamedov, Nazim, N. P. Mehdiyeva, and Lyle E. Craker. "Medicinal Plants Used in Traditional Medicine of the Caucasus and North America." *Journal of Medicinally Active Plants* 4, no. 3 (2015): 42–66. www.doi.org/10.7275/R51834DS.

McGrew, Roderick. *Encyclopedia of Medical History*. New York: McGraw Hill, 1985.

Mességué, Maurice. *Health Secrets of Plants and Herbs*. London: Collins, 1979.

Meyers, Allen. *The Jewish Community of South Philadelphia*. Images of America. Charleston, SC: Arcadia, 1998.

Mills, Simon, and Kerry Bone. *Principles and Practice of Phytotherapy: Modern Herbal Medicine*. Edinburgh, Scotland: Churchill Livingstone, 2000.

Moldenke, Harold N., and Alma L. Moldenke. *Plants of the Bible*. A New Series of Plant Science Books, Vol. 28. Waltham, MA: Chronica Botanica, 1952.

Mokotoff, Gary, and Sallyann Amdur Sack. *Where Once We Walked: A Guide to the Jewish Communities Destroyed in the Holocaust*. Teaneck, NJ: Avotaynu, 1991.

Moskalewicz, Marcin, Ute Caumanns, and Fritz Dross. "Jewish–German–Polish: Histories and Traditions in Medical Culture." In *Jewish Medicine and Healthcare in Central Eastern Europe, Religion, Spirituality and Health: A Social Scientific Approach*, edited by Marcin Moskalewicz, Ute Caumanns, and Fritz Dross, 1–9. Cham, Switzerland: Springer, 2019. www.doi.org/10.1007/978-3-319-92480-9_1.

Mucz, Michael. *Baba's Kitchen Medicines: Folk Remedies of Ukrainian Settlers in Western Canada*. Edmonton: University of Alberta Press, 2012.

Müller-Dietz, Heinz, and Kurt Rintelen. *Arzneipflanzen in der Sowjetunion* [Medicinal plants in the Soviet Union]. Freie Universität. Osteuropa-Institut. Berichte. Reihe Medizin, Folge 18. Berlin, 1960.

Nosal', M. A., and I. M. Nosal'. *Likars'ki Roslyny i Sposoby ikh Zastosuvannia v Narodi* [Medicinal plants and their means of usage among the people]. Kyïv: Vyd-vo "Zdorov'ia," 1964.

Ody, Penelope. *The Complete Medicinal Herbal*. London: Dorling Kindersley, 1993.

Osadcha-Ianata, Nataliia. *Likars'ki roslyny, shcho ïkh uzhyvaje naselennia Pravoberezhnoï Ukraïny v narodnii medycyni* [Medicinal plants as used by populations in Right-Bank Ukraine in folk medicine]. Avgsburg: UVAN, 1949.

Osadcha-Ianata, Nataliia. *Ukraïns'ki narodni nazvy roslyn (zibrav avtor na Ukraïni v rokakh 1927–1939)* [Ukrainian folk names for plants (collected by the author in Ukraine, 1927–1939)]. Niu-Iork: Vydano Ukraïns'koiu vil'noiu akademijeju nauk u SshA, 1973.

Ossadcha-Janata, Natalia. *Herbs Used in Ukrainian Folk Medicine*. East European Fund, Mimeographed Series, No. 21. New York: Research Program on the U.S.S.R. and the New York Botanical Garden, 1952.

Paracelsus, and Arthur Edward Waite. *The Hermetic and Alchemical Writings of Aureolus Philippus Theophrastus Bombast, of Hohenheim, Called Paracelsus the Great*. London: J. Elliott, 1894. www.archive.org/details/hermeticandalch00paragoog.

Patai, Raphael. *On Jewish Folklore*. Detroit: Wayne State University Press, 1983.

Petrovsky-Shtern, Yohanan. "Ba'alei Shem." In *The YIVO Encyclopedia of Jews in Eastern Europe*, edited by Gershon David Hundert, 99–100. New Haven, CT: Yale University Press, 2008.

Petrovsky-Shtern, Yohanan. "Demons." In *The YIVO Encyclopedia of Jews in Eastern Europe*, edited by Gershon David Hundert, 222–23. New Haven, CT: Yale University Press, 2008.

Petrovsky-Shtern, Yohanan. "'You Will Find It in the Pharmacy': Practical Kabbalah and Natural Medicine in Polish Lithuanian Commonwealth, 1690–1750." *Holy Dissent: Jewish and Christian Mystics in Eastern Europe*, edited by Glenn Dynner, 13–53. Detroit: Wayne State University Press, 2011.

Pollack, Herman. *Jewish Folkways in Germanic Lands (1648–1806): Studies in Aspects of Daily Life*. Cambridge, MA: MIT Press, 1971.

Rechtman, Abraham. *Yidishe etnografye un folklor: zikhroynes vegn der etnografisher ekspeditsye, ongefirt fun Sh. An-Ski* [Yiddish ethnography and folklore: memories of the ethnographic expedition led by Sh. An-Sky]. Buenos-Ayres: Yidisher Visnshaftlekher Institut, 1958.

Reid, Daniel P. *Chinese Herbal Medicine*. Boston: Shambhala, 1986.

von Richter, Wilhelm Michael. *Geschichte Der Medicin in Russland* [A history of medicine in Russia]. Moskwa: Wsewolojsky, 1813–1817.

Riddle, John M. *Contraception and Abortion from the Ancient World to the Renaissance*. Cambridge, MA: Harvard University Press, 1992.

Rose, Jeanne. *Herbs & Things: Jeanne Rose's Herbal*. New York: Grosset & Dunlap, 1976.

Roskies, Diane K., and David G. Roskies. *The Shtetl Book*. New York: Ktav Publishing House, 1975.

Rubin, Richard L. "Healing with Plants in Jewish Culture." In *Folk Medicine and Herbal Healing*, edited by George G. Meyer, Kenneth Blum, and John G Cull, 166–75. Springfield, IL: Thomas, 1981.

Safran, Gabriella. *Wandering Soul: The Dybbuk's Creator, S. An-Sky*. Cambridge, MA: Belknap Press of Harvard University Press, 2010.

Schloff, Linda Mack. *And Prairie Dogs Weren't Kosher: Jewish Women in the Upper Midwest Since 1855*. St. Paul: Minnesota Historical Society Press, 1996.

Schulz, Hugo. *Vorlesungen über Wirkung und Anwendung der deutschen Arzneipflanzen* [Lectures on the effects and applications of German medicinal plants]. Leipzig, Germany: Verlag Georg Thieme, 1919.

Schwartz, Joseph. "Tipn un geshtaltn" [Types and figures]. In *Sefer Burshtin*, edited by Shimon Kants, 264–65. Yerushalayim, Tel Aviv: "Entsiklopedyah shel galiut," 1960. www.yiddishbookcenter.org/collections/yizkor-books/yzk-nybc313718.

Seltzer, Leon E. *The Columbia Lippincott Gazetteer of the World*. New York: Columbia University Press, 1952.

Shandler, Jeffrey, and Jonathan Rosen. *Lives Remembered: A Shtetl through a Photographer's Eye.* New York: Museum of Jewish Heritage, 2002.

Shekhṭer, Mortkhe. *Di gevisksn-velt in Yidish* [The plant world in Yiddish]. Nyu-Yorḳ: Yidisher visnshaftllekher institut-YIVO, 2005.

Sidel, Victor W. "Feldshers and 'Feldsherism': The Role and Training of the Feldsher in the USSR." *New England Journal of Medicine* 278, no. 17 (1968): 934–39. www.nejm.org /doi/full/10.1056/NEJM196804252781705.

Suhl, Yuri. *One Foot in America.* New York: Macmillan, 1950.

Theiss, Barbara, and Peter Theiss. *The Family Herbal: A Guide to Natural Health Care for Yourself and Your Children from Europe's Leading Herbalists.* Rev. ed. Rochester, VT: Healing Arts Press, 1993.

Tissot, S. A. D. *Advice to the People in General with Regard to Their Health: But More Particularly Calculated for Those Who, by Their Distance from Regular Physicians or Other Very Experienced Practitioners, Are the Most Unlikely to Be Seasonably Provided with the Best Advice and Assistance in Acute Diseases, or upon Any Sudden Inward or Outward Accident: With a Table of the Most Cheap, Yet Effectual Remedies, and the Plainest Directions for Preparing Them Readily.* Translated by J. Kirkpatrick. London: Printed for T. Becket and P. A. De Hondt, 1765. www.gutenberg.org/files/39044/39044-h/39044-h.htm.

Trachtenberg, Joshua. *Jewish Magic and Superstition: A Study in Folk Religion.* New York: Behrman's Jewish Book House, 1939.

Tsherniak, F. "Meditsinishe hilf un meditsinishe anshtaltn" [Medical aid and medical establishments]. In *Antopolye: Sefer-yizkor*, edited by Benzion Ayalon, 527–33. Steven Spielberg Digital Yiddish Library, No. 13678. Amherst, MA: National Yiddish Book Center, 2001. www.yiddishbookcenter.org/collections/yizkor-books/yzk-nybc313678.

Tuszewicki, Marek. "German Medicine, Folklore and Language in Popular Medical Practices of the Eastern European Jews (Nineteenth to Twentieth Century)." In *Jewish Medicine and Healthcare in Central Eastern Europe, Religion, Spirituality and Health: A Social Scientific Approach*, edited by Marcin Moskalewicz, Ute Caumanns, and Fritz Dross, 63–78. Cham, Switzerland: Springer, 2019. www.doi.org/10.1007/978-3-319-92480-9_5.

Tuviah ha-Rofe (Tobias Cohn, Tobias ha-Kohen). *Ma'aseh Tuviah* [The work of Tobias]. Krakow, Poland, 1908.

Vasiliauskas, Juozas. *Vaistažolių Galia* [The power of herbal medicine]. Vilnius, Lithuania: Politika, 1991.

Vogl, Sylvia, Paolo Picker, Judit Mihaly-Bison, Nanang Fakhrudin, Atanas G. Atanasov, Elke H. Heiss, Christoph Wawrosch, Reznicek Gottfried, Verena M. Dirsch, Johannes Saukel, and Brigitte Kopp. "Ethnopharmacological in vitro Studies on Austria's Folk Medicine—An Unexplored Lore: In vitro Anti-Inflammatory Activities of 71 Austrian Traditional

Herbal Drugs." *Journal of Ethnopharmacology* 149, no. 3 (2013): 750–71. www.doi
.org/10.1016/j.jep.2013.06.007.

Warburg, Otto. *Die Muskatnuss: Ihre Geschichte, Botanik, Kultur, Handel Und Verwerthung
Sowie Ihre Verfälschungen Und Surrogate: Zugleich Ein Beitrag Zur Kulturgeschichte
Der Banda-Inseln* [Nutmeg: its history, botany, culture, trade, and use, as well as its adul-
terations and substitutes: being at the same time a cultural history of the Banda Islands].
Leipzig, Germany: W. Engelmann, 1897.

Wengeroff, Pauline, and Shulamit S. Magnus. *Memoirs of a Grandmother: Scenes from the
Cultural History of the Jews of Russia in the Nineteenth Century.* 2 vols. Stanford, CA:
Stanford University Press, 2010.

Wheelwright, Edith Grey. *Medicinal Plants and Their History.* New York: Dover, 1974.

Wood, George B., Franklin Bache, H. C. Wood, Joseph P. Remington, and Samuel P. Sadtler.
The Dispensatory of the United States of America. Philadelphia: Lippincott, 1918.

Woodhead, Lindy. *War Paint: Madame Helena Rubinstein and Miss Elizabeth Arden: Their
Lives, Their Times, Their Rivalry.* Hoboken, NJ: John Wiley & Sons, 2003.

Wu, Jing-Nuan. *An Illustrated Chinese Materia Medica.* New York: Oxford University Press,
2005.

Zborowski, Mark, Elizabeth Herzog, and Margaret Mead. *Life Is with People: The Culture of
the Shtetl.* New York: Schocken Books, 1962.

Zemlinskii, S. E. *Lekarstvennye Rasteniia SSSR* [Medicinal plants of the USSR]. Izd. 3-e ispr.
i doped. Moskva: Medgiz, 1958.

Zevin, Igor Vilevich, Nathaniel Altman, and Lilia Vasilevna Zevin. *A Russian Herbal: Traditional Remedies for Health and Healing.* Rochester, VT: Healing Arts Press, 1997.

Zimmels, Hirsch Jacob. *Magicians, Theologians and Doctors: Studies in Folk-Medicine
and Folk-Lore as Reflected in the Rabbinical Responsa (12th–19th Centuries).* London:
Edward Goldston, 1952.

Zinberg, Israel. *The Berlin Haskalah.* A History of Jewish Literature, Vol. 8. Cincinnati, OH:
Hebrew Union College Press, 1976.

INDEX

Chemist and Druggist publication, 223
chicken pox, nettle for, 243
chicken soup, 55
chicken soup theory, 2
chicory. *See Cichorium intybus* (chicory)
chilblains
defined, 267
horsetail for, 110
mallow for, 145
childbirth
delphinium for, 105, 106
dropwort for, 121
horsetail for hemorrhaging, 112
mallow for, 144–145
nettle for after, 240
pepperwort for speedy, 153
Potentilla for, 199
raspberry for, 210, 211, 213
Trifolium for complications after, 234
water lily increases lactation after, 168
white peony for, 172
children
chicory for ailments of, 95
knotweed for thrush or nettle rash, 190
mallow for teething, 145
meadowsweet for diarrhea, 118
nettle for eczema, 241
nutmeg for diarrhea, 161–162
peony for teething, 173
plantago for bone fractures, 184
plantago for dysentery, 182
St. John's wort for bedwetting, 134
St. John's wort for diarrhea, 139
violet for epilepsy, 249
white peony for epilepsy, 176
wild strawberry for cough and colds, 129
cholagogue
chelidonium as, 84
defined, 266
Lepidium as, 153
Trifolium as, 229
cholera
knotweed for, 186, 187
wormwood for, 79
choleretic, 84, 266

cholesterol, 92, 241
cicatrisant, 266
Cichorium intybus (chicory)
common names, 89–90
in contemporary herbalism, 91–92
description and location of, 90
early remedies, 90–91
in early twentieth century Europe, 92–94
in the Pale in early twentieth century, 94–96
cinquefoil. *See Potentilla anserina*
circulation
comfrey for, 223
Lepidium for, 153
nettle for, 240, 244
nutmeg for, 160
civilian barber-surgeons, 14
Claudius Galenus. *See* Galen
Clusius, Carolus, 83
clyster
defined, 266
mallow prepared as, 144
plantago prepared as, 178
coagulant, horsetail as, 109–110
cobwebs
bandaging minor cuts with fresh, 63
preventing gangrene, 15–16
treating boils, 29
coffee
roasted acorns as substitute for, 204–205
roasted chicory mixed with, 92–93
water lily *as* substitute for, 169
Cohn, Tobias. *See* ha-Kohen, Tobias
colds
comfrey for, 224
Cynoglossum for, 98–100
dropwort for, 121
horsetail for, 112
knotweed for, 190
mallow for, 147, 149
meadowsweet for, 118
nettle for, 244–245
plantago for, 180, 183
raspberry for, 211–212

ACKNOWLEDGMENTS

WE WOULD LIKE TO THANK the following libraries and archives for their invaluable assistance throughout this project, including the staff of the Ukrainian Free Academy of Sciences (UVAN) in New York and the staff of Columbia University's Special Collections Department for their aid and assistance. We would particularly like to acknowledge the Interlibrary Loan Department at UC Davis's Shields Library for locating and delivering so many hard-to-find and hard-to-read sources: many thanks to Jason Newborn, Susan Sullivan, Karen Jones, and Rebecca Moore-Poe for their digilence and hard work. We would also like to thank fellow librarians Daniel Goldstein, Leyla Cabugos, and Axel Borg for their insights, suggestions, and encouragement.

In the herbalist community, we would like to thank Susan Marynowski for recognizing a diamond in the rough and shepherding the first version of this tale into press for the *Journal of the American Herbalists Guild,* and much gratitude to Shayna Keyles and everyone at NAB for believing in this project. We would also like to thank the teachers and students (especially Pamela Fischer) at the Berkeley Herbal Center for building a community and our education. Many thanks to Kendra Marcus for guidance and her faith in this project. Much love and gratitude to our friends: Josh Jones for his secret plant knowledge; Laurie Lee for her sharp-eyed readings of the rocky first drafts; classmates Julia Braun for her chicken soup observation; Kalpana Jacob, Sami Graf, and Yunnie Snyder for encouraging us to untangle this tale; and Autumn Summers for suggesting we pursue publication. Much love and gratitude to our family (especially Nathanael), and we dedicate this book to the memory of our ancestors and, of course, the plants.

ABOUT THE AUTHORS

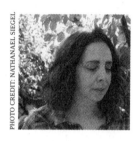

DEATRA COHEN is an author, herbalist, master gardener, and artist. She holds degrees from the University of California, Davis, San Jose State University, and the Berkeley Herbal Center. Deatra lives in Northern California.

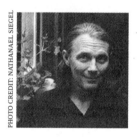

ADAM SIEGEL is an author, translator, and bibliographer. He is a graduate of the University of Minnesota, the University of California, Berkeley, and San Jose State University and lives in Northern California.

About North Atlantic Books

North Atlantic Books (NAB) is a 501(c)(3) nonprofit publisher committed to a bold exploration of the relationships between mind, body, spirit, culture, and nature. Founded in 1974, NAB aims to nurture a holistic view of the arts, sciences, humanities, and healing. To make a donation or to learn more about our books, authors, events, and newsletter, please visit www.northatlanticbooks.com.